Forest Dragon Exercises

林龍功

Forest Dragon Exercises

林龍功

Phase I

An Introduction to the Forest Dragon System of Pai Lum

Nian-Li Pai

J G Lynn

Nian Media

Nian Brands Corporation

Wilmington, Delaware

ISBN   978-0692692219

     (0692692215)

First Edition

林龍功

Lin Long Kung

www.ForestDragon.org

Table of Contents

Forest Dragon Exercises

Preface

I began studying Pai Lum in 1974 under John A. Weninger, who I would come to know as Pai Li Lung, my teacher for forty-two years. Later that same year I trained for the first time with his teacher, Grandmaster Daniel K. Pai, at a clinic, the first of many over the next twenty years with one of the most renowned and skilled practitioners of the twentieth century.

Shortly after I began training I decided that I wanted not only to excel in this art but that I wanted to be a part of teaching it to others. In 1975 I was accepted into the Student Instructor Trainee course, an intensive training program taught by Pai Li Lung and his top level instructors. I have been teaching Pai Lum ever since.

After twenty-five years of teaching I began to see the need for a highly-focused system of exercises, techniques, and sequences that would convey the core concepts of Pai Lum. I had seen that for many people it was becoming more difficult to commit a significant amount of time to learn and practice martial arts. While I still believe it is preferable for students to attend classes at least twice a week and train at least an hour a day, I realized that there were some that would never be able to commit to this level of training and might be denied the benefits of martial arts training.

In the summer of 2000 I decided to begin developing the Forest Dragon Exercises. My goal was to create a system of exercises specifically designed to promote health and well-being without requiring a large time commitment. At the same time I wanted to introduce the key concepts of the combative arts more commonly known as *Chinese kung fu.*

iii

Over the past 10 years I continually worked to refine the exercises. I eventually formalized this system into five groups of exercises which I refer to as the five phases of development in the lower levels of Pai Lum. The first of these phases is presented in this book.

Although the Forest Dragon Exercises are completely my own, they draw heavily on everything I have learned in Pai Lum in over forty years. Many of the techniques are taken directly from the traditional sets we train. All of this is possible due to the countless hours spent with my teacher Pai Li Lung along with Grandmaster Pai and countless other masters who were frequent guests at our training sessions. I would also like to thank my good friend and fellow Pai Lum practitioner Kirk Kozero for all of the feedback he gave me while writing this book.

Nian Li Pai
J G Lynn

4 July, 2016

The art is truth: truth is the art.
It knows nothing of any name we might give it.
It recognizes no masters.

The art flows like a river
from practitioner to practitioner,
from generation to generation,
constantly changing yet always the same art.

Those who follow it keep it alive, and the art them.
The art dismisses those who have no use for it
and it no use for them.
It will always be the art:
no more — no less.

- Nian-li Pai (J G Lynn)

Introduction

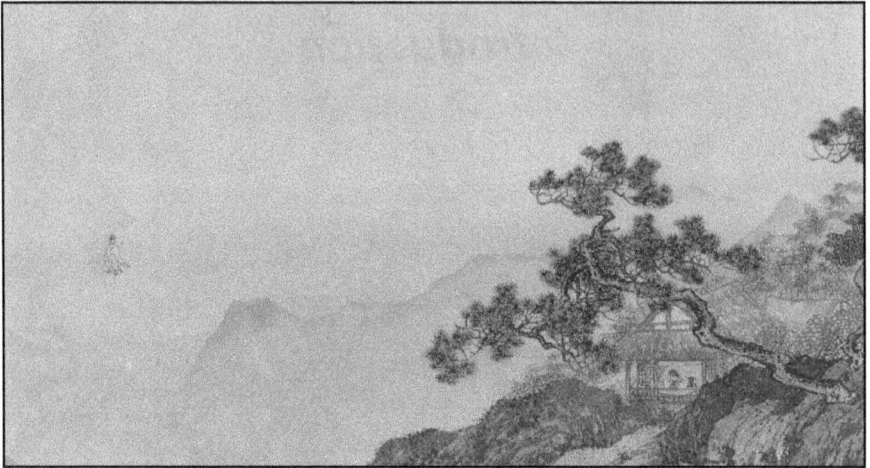

Dreaming of Immortality, T'ang Yin, Ming Dynasty

For centuries, civilizations have dreamed of immortality. Ancient cultures from China to Egypt have strived to prolong their lifespan or even to avoid death completely. There are countless manuscripts describing methods of purifying the body in an effort to evade this ultimate fate. Legends have emerged of masters who withdrew from civilization to live a life of isolation in pursuit of this elusive goal. Perhaps the most famous of these was a Chinese martial artist and herbalist by the name of Lǐ Qīngyún who lived to the age of 197, although some claimed he was actually 256 when he died in 1933.

Certainly there are many factors that may contribute to a prolonged lifespan and many factors that will shorten it. A good diet and regular exercise combined with a healthy lifestyle are key to a long life and a life worth living. By providing a structure of daily exercise, the Forest Dragon Exercises attempt to make life better and longer for anyone who cares to practice them.

This book is a training manual and a reference for students, which will provide a reference for the student. No book can serve as a replacement for a qualified teacher. There are many qualified teachers of Pai Lum, including the instructors of the Forest Dragon School. The principles of exercise, training, and human physiology are the same regardless of the method of training employed. Therefore, any qualified teacher will be able to use this book as a tool to be used as an aid in training.

Some of the exercises in this book are derived directly from yoga. The postures have been adapted to fit specific purposes and may not always reflect the way they might be practiced in any particular school of yoga, but they closely resemble the original yogic posture and in many cases are identical. Where applicable, the names for the yoga postures are provided on the right side of the page in both English and Sanskrit as a reference. Although it is not necessary to learn the Sanskrit names for the postures or the yogic methods, some may find it interesting to know more about the historic origins of

3

these exercises, which are thousands of years old, perhaps the oldest exercises still practiced today.

There are many systems of physical exercise and many have been developed for specific purposes. Some are developed specifically to develop one's ability as a golfer or a fighter. People who want to be a champion swimmer or a professional football player may have a personal trainer who coaches them on how best to increase the specific skills necessary for that sport, focusing on maximizing their strength, developing muscle tone and speed, or developing their endurance.

Pai Lum focuses on all of these and it focuses on none of these. We develop strength but don't focus on it. We develop endurance but don't focus on it. The same is true of flexibility, speed, and coordination. It is left to the individual to focus on whatever is important to them.

What is Pai Lum?

Pai Lum is not a specific set of exercises or movements – it is a way of moving. It is not characterized by one technique or another – it is a way of fighting. Pai Lum is a way of thinking – a way of living. This is the essence of Pai Lum.

Pai Li Lung gave the following answer to the question "What is Pai Lum?"

To answer this question in a few short sentences is almost impossible. It may even take a book full of writing to do the definition justice. But in any event, I shall try.

The thoughts and definitions contained herein are my personal feelings, and understandings based on my personal journey through Pai Lum.

Pai Lum is a martial art.

Pai Lum is a way of life.

Pai Lum is a self defense.

Pai Lum is a philosophy.

Pai Lum is an exercise.

Pai Lum is nature.

Gee, maybe it won't take a book full of writing!

For the beginner (first ten years of training) one should focus entirely on basics. This includes basic fighting techniques, theories, and concepts, basic health techniques, both internal, external, and the basic philosophy of Pai Lum.

A beginner should learn how to construct the basic techniques, the mechanics of executing the techniques, and the basic striking points on which to apply the techniques. This method of learning may appear to be slow, but a good understanding of the purpose and function of techniques is essential for the mind to accept that technique and allow it to work.

Pai Lum for the beginner starts with practice and repetition. In order for the mind to accept and understand a technique, it must be thoroughly familiar with that technique. It must be friends with it. It must know it as one knows the neighborhood one grew up in; all the back alleys and shortcuts, where to go and where no to go.

When the mind gets this familiar with a technique, it accepts it and uses it without thinking when the need arises.

So remember, what the mind accepts, the body must do.

And this is accomplished through:

> *Repetition*

> *Repetition*

> *Repetition*

I always tell my students that when they become sick and tired of doing a technique, they are probably beginning to master it, and their real training is just beginning. It is essential to master your basics because advanced Pai Lum is basics combined and applied without thinking as a situation calls for it.

Now, since we realize that there is a lot of physical practice for the beginner, we must also realize that the philosophy of Pai Lum is found through that physical training. The motions and positions cause the mind to see and understand the true nature of being and why things are the way they are.

Truth is not what someone tells you it is. It is what it is. This becomes apparent throughout the physical practice of Pai Lum.

I would like to interject a thought at this point. I believe Pai Lum to be a unique and individual art that is not like any other. Sometimes it might appear to be similar to other arts, but that is usually an intentional illusion; "illusion structure"as Lung would say. It has a deeper truth to it and causes each practitioner to be able to make it work in their own way, quite unusual and hard to explain if you haven't experienced it. That is what Grandmaster Pai brought to the students, and this is why they may do the same technique, but appear to be different. Pai Lum is not a technique, it is a way of doing technique.

In order for Pai Lum to continue for the next generations, it must rise above any individual. To do that, the responsibility is given to me by Lung, I have established a system of progressive learning.

It starts at the very beginning, and slowly takes a student on a journey towards mastering this art in an orderly and reasonable manner.

Things are learned when they should be learned, not before or after. You start at the beginning and continue to add things to your learning so that you progress smoothly from beginner, to intermediate, to advanced level until you simply realize you are a practitioner of Pai Lum.

Forest Dragon Exercises

There are no tests, sashes, or titles. The only exception is in teaching. You must be given permission to instruct by your teacher and license to teach by your teacher.

I believe that the true study of Pai Lum is to reach a level of "egolessness". How can we do this if ego-promoting ranks and titles are used? It may look good on paper, but in application, it does not seem to work Grandmaster Pai said "I do not call myself a master", neither should we. If someone recognizes your achievements, and acknowledges them by calling you by a title, the humility learned in practice should cause you to continue training and not go on an ego trip. In other words, I know how much I don't know. Remember, skill is relative. A beginner might think you are a master, but your teacher thinks you need more work and practice. It's relative to who's watching you.

There was an old Tai Chi master who would cry whenever he did his form. When asked why, he said, "I've been doing this for 70 years, and it's still not right." So let us not think we are that good, we still need improvement. If you are a senior, humbly help those under you, don't gloat in your achievements and you will truly be masterful.

Now, on with the Journey!

About This Book

Over the past 100 years the world has changed greatly. We enjoy many improvements to our life, but it does not come without a cost – greater distractions and less time. Most people today do not have the time to dedicate long hours of practice to learn and master the martial arts or even to adhere to a regular exercise regimen. I began developing the exercises that I call Forest Dragon exercises in 2000 to introduce students to the fundamentals of Pai Lum Kung Fu using a core set of exercises and techniques which can be practiced daily in a small amount of time. Needless to say, the more time one can devote to exercise and practice, the better the results and the more proficient they will become.

This book is the first in a series of five which contains all of the fundamental exercises, including breathing exercises, yoga postures, stances, basic kicks, strikes, and blocks in the form of fighting sequences which will give a student everything he needs to begin the practice of Pai Lum.

Many people ask whether Pai Lum is a "hard" style or a "soft" style. Japanese and Okinawan karate are examples of hard styles because of the crisp, linear movements. Many Chinese styles, but not all, are considered soft styles due to their circular movements which gives them a softer appearance. The beginning phases of Pai Lum Kung Fu are made up of what many people today call Kenpo, or Kempo, or *quan fa* in Chinese. Quan fa means "way of the fist", "law of the fist", or just simply "fist way". Quan fa can be regarded as the basics of kung fu, which will become evident in this first book, phase one of the Forest Dragon exercises.

Forest Dragon Exercises

In the next three phases, the student will be introduced to
concepts which go beyond the more simple principles and in
the fifth phase the student is introduced to the basic concepts
of tai chi. Tai chi represents the other end of the spectrum
from quan fa. It can be regarded as the final phase of an
introduction to Pai Lum, which is to say the student is finally
well on their way to a lifetime of learning.

The intent of this book is not to replace the teacher, but to
provide a tool which can be used as a reference for the
student. This book assumes that the student has a qualified
instructor to teach them the correct execution of stances,
punches, kicks, and other techniques. The movements and
sequences can be learned without a teacher if the aim is to
gain the benefits to one's physical and mental health. This will
provide a basis which can be built upon by a teacher for those
who may wish to continue their study of kung fu more
seriously and gain a better understanding of Pai Lum and its
combative aspects.

Students often ask which style of martial art is best or whether
one school is better than another. There is an old adage in the
martial arts,
>   "There are many paths which lead to the top of the
>   mountain. Whichever path you take, the view at the top
>   is the same."

It is true that there is no single path that is better than the rest;
however, not all paths lead to the top of the mountain. Some
paths lead in the wrong direction – away from the top of the
mountain. And some paths lead deep into the forest where
you will remain – lost forever. Whichever path you may
choose, find a teacher who will keep you on the right path and
help you find your way upward.

A Brief History of Martial Arts

Forest Dragon Exercises

Martial arts exist in all parts of the world. This book focuses on martial arts which originated in Asia. Many, but not all, Asian martial arts trace their roots to China. Popular martial arts such as Japanese karate, Okinawan kempo, and Korean taekwondo were derived directly from Chinese arts.

Although historical records describing the Chinese martial arts go back over 4,000 years to the Yellow Emperor, Huángdì, most modern styles of kung fu are derived from the martial practices of the Buddhist monks at the Shaolin temple. The origin of Shaolin kung fu can be traced back to Bhodidharma, the 28th patriarch of Buddha, who is credited with bringing Chan Buddhism from India to China somewhere between 523 and 527 AD. Upon arriving at Shaolin he found the monks to be in poor health. He taught them how to better take care of themselves through herbal medicine, diet, and exercise. These exercises included internal exercises known as Sinew Changing exercises and an external exercise set known as the Eighteen Hands of Arhat. The term external refers to the emphasis on the development of the muscles and external movements. Internal exercises emphasize the development of breathing and internal energy. These external exercises are what were developed over the next 1000 years into what has become known today as Shaolin kung fu. Somewhere around the 13th century one of Shaolin's best practitioners, Chueh Yuan, sought out Li Sou, another well-known practitioner, along with Pai Yu-feng. The three of them returned to Shaolin where they spent several years developing Shaolin kung fu into a set of 170 techniques that formed the basis for modern Shaolin kung fu.

Over the centuries the Shaolin system evolved. Many of the practitioners who left the monastery or who studied there went on to develop their own styles.. Many of these styles were only taught to members of the family and as a result, many ceased to exist when the last practicing family member died without passing their style on to a successor. One of the family styles which survived is Pai Lum.

History of Pai Lum

As a family style, Pai Lum was only taught to members of the Pai family. Pai Lum kung fu is a term used by the founder of the system, Grandmaster Daniel K. Pai, to refer to his teachings. Grandmaster Pai was a Chinese-Hawaiian who was taught by his grandfather, who had his own name for the system. Although the Pai family system has been handed down from generation to generation, it has been the tradition for each generation to change the name used to refer to the teachings. The system's name reflects the generation or family member who taught it. When his grandfather died, the grandmaster title and the system passed to the next practicing relative, and the system was given the name Pai Lum.

The Chinese characters for the system's name actually translate literally as "white dragon skilled man". But, like many Chinese terms, this one has many meanings, references, and definitions. "Pai" means "white" or "pure". It also is the surname of grandmaster Daniel K. Pai. "Lum" is Cantonese for "forest" which symbolizes unknown knowledge. Kung fu is the generic term used in the United States to refer to the Chinese martial arts. It means skilled man or skill achieved through time and effort. A skilled flower arranger, dancer, or astronaut has kung fu. Pai Lum therefore, means White Forest and Pai Lum Kung Fu can be loosely translated as "a person who is skilled in pure knowledge." There are more meanings to the name, some of which are deeper, more symbolic, or special to the Pai family of practitioners.

Upon the death of Grandmaster Daniel K. Pai, the Pai Lum system was passed to his senior student, John A Weninger, who had been given the name Li Lung Pai. In order to preserve the tradition of teaching the family style only to members of the Pai family, Grandmaster Pai had begun granting his top students the status of "adopted grandchildren" and giving them a Pai family name.

The martial arts training of Li Lung Pai started back in 1964, when he began studying Judo, the gentle way. Shortly after her took up judo, he began studying Shorin-Ryu Karate. His training, however, was interrupted when he was called upon to serve his country in the U.S. Army.

Upon returning home to Bethlehem, PA where he was born and raised, he searched out his Judo instructor who was now teaching Japanese-style Karate. Li Lung enrolled in the school and after about two and a half years was promoted to Shodan,

Note that the family name sometimes comes first and other times comes last. For example, you may see either Pai Li Lung or Li Lung Pai. This is because in Chinese the family name always comes first. In western cultures the family name is the last name. Although many of us within Pai Lum prefer the traditional rendition, it is less confusing for people in the west to put the family name last. For this reason I have chosen to use the latter in this book.

First Degree Black Belt. By this time he had opened his own school in Allentown, PA and immediately after his promotion he established his second school in Bethlehem. One year later Li Lung opened a third school in Quakertown, PA. Realizing he could no longer manage more schools himself he began to franchise his schools under the name of Weninger Karate Institute and opened a fourth school in Scranton, PA. Over the next several years he continued to grow across Pennsylvania.

In the meantime, Li Lung Pai continued his studies in the martial arts with an instructor who trained him in Chinese Kempo and he soon received his Second Degree Black Belt. He also trained in Aikido, Judo, and various weapons. It was after his instructor decided to go his own way that Li Lung met Daniel K. Pai who introduced him to Pai Lum Kung Fu. He was accepted as a student of Grand Master Pai and was soon made a Disciple. Not long after that Grand Master Pai made him an adopted grandson and gave him his Chinse name – Li Lung Pai, an honor Li Lung said he would spend the rest of his life trying to live up to.

Over the next several decades Li Lung continued to train with Grand Master Pai. He also allowed hundreds of his own students to benefit directly from Grand Master Pai's teaching by hosting many seminars with the Grand Master as well as summer training camps with classes in various styles of martial arts taught by some of the most prestigious martial artists in the U.S.

When asked to describe himself as a martial artist, Li Lung Pai replied, "I am a practitioner of Kung Fu. Totally dedicated and involved in my art. I am a guide to my students, so they may learn, and I am always in search of new knowledge so I may better myself as a human being and in turn, better my brothers."

After Grandmaster Pai's death in 1993, Li Lung Pai became the head of the Pai Lum family and began adopting the next generation of grandchildren. Because Grandmaster Pai was Chinese-Hawaiian, Li Lung decided to give us names that were part Chinese and part Hawaiian. I was adopted into the Pai family as Nalu Li Pai, which translates to Nian Li Pai when written in Chinese characters.

Forest Dragon Exercises

Practice of Forest Dragon Exercises

Forest Dragon Exercises

How to Train

Training with Grandmaster Pai was always interesting, sometimes difficult, and we never knew what to expect. No matter what he was teaching he was able to keep everyone's attention. He never seemed to take anything too seriously and yet everyone took him very seriously. He often interjected things like "Don't look so serious", or "put a smile on your face, you'll be going home soon." Even when he was demonstrating how to destroy an opponent he liked to say, "Have a good time." I have learned that this is important when training. It should always be enjoyable. If you aren't having a good time, you should find something else to do. Life's too short to spend it practicing something that is a chore.

So just what should you practice? Li Lung Pai said, "Pai Lum for the beginner starts with practice and repetition." Almost a hundred years earlier another great master, Gichin Funakoshi, wrote,

> *"Although karate can be easily memorized, it can be easily forgotten as well; thus, once a kata is memorized, it must be repeated again and again. Like water, heat must be added to the boiling pot of water lest it return to its cold water state."*

The more a student practices the better they will become. But repetition alone is not sufficient. It is more productive to practice a kick or a strike ten times with full attention to the technique, being fully mindful of executing the best technique possible, than it is to practice one hundred or even one thousand times in a half-hearted manner without engaging mentally in the training at hand.

Likewise, the length of time a student practices is not as important as how often they practice. The goal should be to practice daily. Ten minutes every day is better for learning than two hours once each week. Naturally, I would encourage everyone to devote more than 5 minutes each day if at all possible. Each student should set their own personal minimums according to their schedule and do their best to commit to those minimums.

At the end of this book I will lay out an approach to training the Forest Dragon exercises in ways that can fit into any schedule – even ten minutes.

Lastly, do not leave training in the training hall. Think of your everyday life as martial arts training. Look for opportunities throughout every day to practice and apply what you learn, whether it is simply the way you breathe, the way you stand, or the way you move from one place to another. Allow the concepts you learn during your formal training to expand into everything you do. The effect can be surprising.

One thing the student should always remember is to maintain a deep regard for courtesy, and to be respectful to one's seniors. All martial arts stress the importance of courtesy and respect. After all, learning a martial art is not about learning to fight, it is about learning to live. It's not just about how to survive but how to get along with the rest of the world.

Breaking

Breaking boards, bricks, and other materials has become an inseparable part of the martial arts. This is understandable; it can be very impressive to watch, and it is a lot of fun! But why do we break boards, bricks, cement blocks, or any other object? Breaking is a tool, one of many, to understand our capabilities. It helps us understand if a technique is effective and helps us build confidence. Unfortunately, too much emphasis is put on this aspect of training and those who do not practice the martial arts themselves often view it as proof of mastery.

Five Elements

In traditional Chinese philosophy, many things are classified into five elements. The elements are earth, metal, water, wood, and fire. The elements are tied together in a 'cycle' of creation, sometimes called the cycle of generation. Earth gives rise to metal, metal gives rise to water, water gives rise to wood, and wood gives rise to fire. The traditional theory of the five elements was a metaphysical attempt at explaining the world and everything in it. Therefore, the concepts in the cycle of creation and the cycle of destruction are found throughout traditional Chinese martial arts theory, particularly the internal styles. These traditional arts often explain the manipulation of energy inside the human body in terms of the five elements.

The five phases of the Forest Dragon Exercises are referred to as Young Dragon, Inner Dragon, Outer Dragon, Flying Dragon, and Ancient Dragon. Each phase corresponds to one of the elements and the progression through the phases corresponds to the cycle of creation.

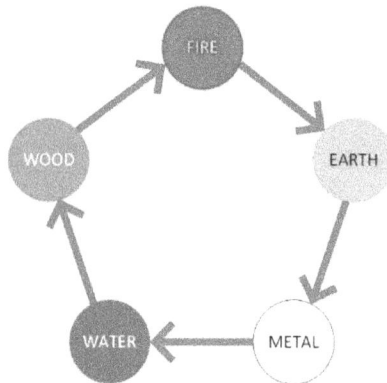

FIRE

WOOD

EARTH

WATER

METAL

The five phases are used to give the set of exercises structure. This structure makes it easier to learn the exercises and the concepts behind them in a more natural and deliberate progression. The exercises are divided into five phases through which the student progresses, each associated with one of the elements. Each phase also introduces a sequence known as a movement form. The names of these forms correspond to each of the five phases: Young Dragon, Inner Dragon, Outer Dragon, Flying Dragon, and Ancient Dragon.

- *Earth* is considered the starting point, the ground level so to speak. *Earth* is also associated with the center in Chinese element theory and is associated with the color yellow. In this level of training the student is introduced to the most fundamental exercises, concepts, and theories.

- *Metal* is the next level of training and can be thought of as a refinement of earth, just as metals are mined from the earth and refined. *Metal* is associated with the west in element theory and the color white.

- **Water** follows from metal and introduces the concept of fluidity. The concepts in this level of training focus on flowing motions with particular emphasis on the concept of yielding over that of resistance. *Water* is associated with 'north' and the color grey or black.

- *Wood* From the nourishment of water comes wood. Wood is the only element that is living. It changes as it grows and goes in many directions. This level emphasizes adaptability. *Wood* is associated with east and the color green.

25

- *Fire* is the final element. It is composed more of energy than it is of matter. This level emphasizes the efficient use of energy and is an introduction to the more advanced levels. In this level an explicit differentiation is made between the inner and outer methods of expressing energy. *Fire* is associated with south and the color red.

In addition to the cycle of creation described above, Chinese element theory also describes the cycle of destruction (or restraining cycle). In this cycle, the elements counteract or restrain each other. The cycle of destruction is reflected in the training phases of the higher level student. In order for the student to understand and benefit from the cycle of destruction (or decomposition as I prefer to call it), the principles of the cycle of creation must first be understood.

And now, as Grandmaster Pai Li Lung said, "On with the journey!" And of course – Have a good time!

Meditation, Qi Kung, and Yoga

Forest Dragon Exercises

All students begin training with exercises that prepare them for exercising both the mind and the body. These serve both to warm up and also as conditioning. These exercises are comprised of meditation, qi kung, and yoga. All three are related and there is a great deal of overlap between them.

In Pai Lum, meditation focuses primarily on exercising the mind. Training in Pai Lum begins with the mind and is expressed through physical movements. These movements are what most people think of when they think of kung fu or any other martial art. But the movements differ from many other forms of exercise in the way they are performed. With many exercise routines the emphasis is on performing repetitions of simple movements to develop the muscles. In martial arts there is an emphasis on being mindful of the movements, of beings acutely aware of the movements. The focus proceeds from the mind to the body. For this reason I refer to Pai Lum as an *expressionist* art.

Qi kung can be translated as *breath exercise*. It is closely related and similar to the *pranayama* of yoga. Various aspects of yoga are incorporated into the Forest Dragon exercises to develop flexibility, strength, and health. Pai Lum makes use of many of the benefits of yoga. Further background on yoga can be found in the back of the book.

Breathing and Meditation

Earth Breathing

Earth Breathing is the fundamental breathing technique used in the Forest Dragon Exercises and is the basis for all other breathing exercises. Like most breathing exercises in yoga, qi kung, and martial arts, the main focus is on developing abdominal breathing.

Breathing is nothing more than bringing air into the lungs and then pushing the air back out of the lungs. The most efficient way to pull air into the lungs is by using the diaphragm, a muscle which lies just under the lungs. When the diaphragm contracts it is pulled lower, expanding the lungs at the same time. When the muscle is relaxed, it returns to its resting position allowing the lungs to contract, expelling the air.

The best way to learn the basic technique of abdominal breathing is to begin by lying flat on your back with hands comfortably at the sides and feet slightly apart. Close the eyes and the mouth. Slowly inhale through the nose, drawing the air in deeply but in a natural manner. Exhale through the nose. While inhaling, the lower abdomen should rise, keeping the back relaxed. During the exhalation, the stomach should fall back towards the ground. Breathing should be natural, not forced or exaggerated.

To help develop a good sense of abdominal breathing, visualize your stomach rising and falling. You can get a good feel for this by actually placing something on your stomach and focus on lifting it as high as you can when you inhale as shown in the first picture.

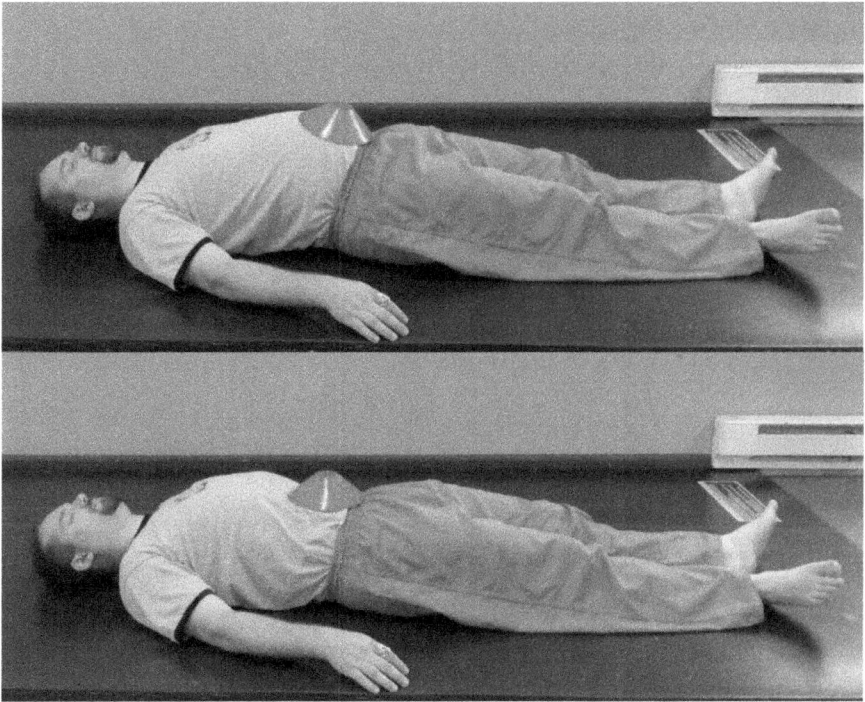

While exhaling you should focus on allowing the object to fall back down, gently pulling the stomach in with the abdominal muscles as shown in the second picture. Allow the rate of breathing to adjust itself. Try to avoid counting or timing the breaths to reach a specific number of breaths per minute.

31

This basic form of breathing is an introduction to meditation as well. Meditation is nothing more than a way of exercising the mind, of making the mind stronger. Concentrating on the breath is a simple way of focusing the mind, of developing the mind's ability to minimize distractions by focusing on a single thought or task. By performing the earth breathing exercise every day you will not only be developing healthier breathing habits, you will be developing your ability to be mindful, to focus on tasks while minimizing mental distraction. This is the first of many meditation techniques utilized in training the mind.

Qi Kung Exercises

Heaven and Earth   (*Tadasana*)

This exercise is very basic yet fundamental to understanding posture and balance. It is related to the yoga posture known as mountain pose or tadasana. In addition to developing a sense of balance, it strengthens the calf, ankle, and foot muscles while stretching the spine and shoulders.

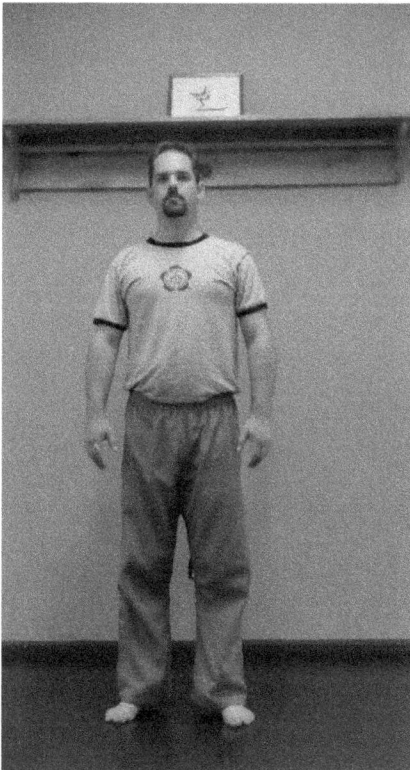

1. Begin standing with the feet a comfortable distance apart, between 6 and 12 inches.

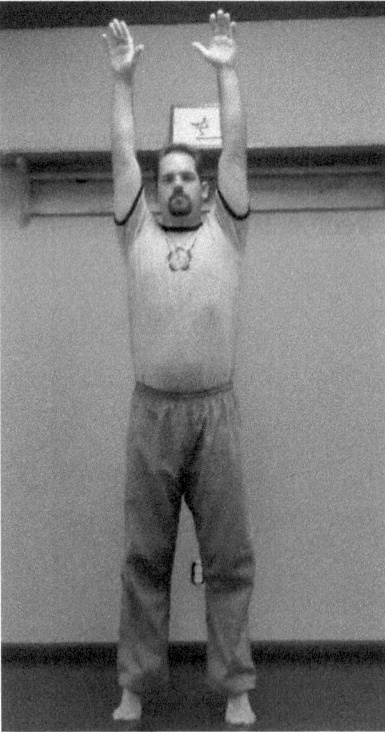

2. Extend the hands and arms upward, palms facing forward, inhaling as you do.

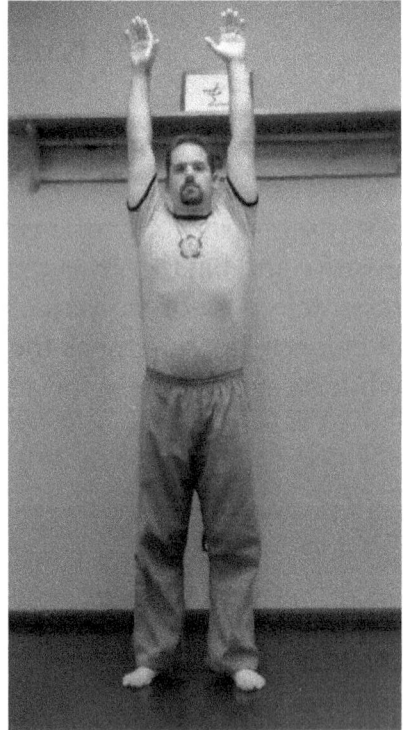

3. Continue extending the hands upward as you raise the heels off of the ground.

4. Reverse the movement and return to the starting position.

Dancing Dragon (*Natarajasana*)

This exercise focuses on balance while stretching the quadriceps, the top thigh muscle, and the ligaments.

1. From a standing position, begin by raising one leg behind you, grasping with one hand.

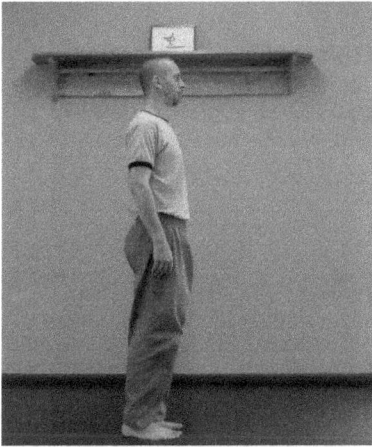

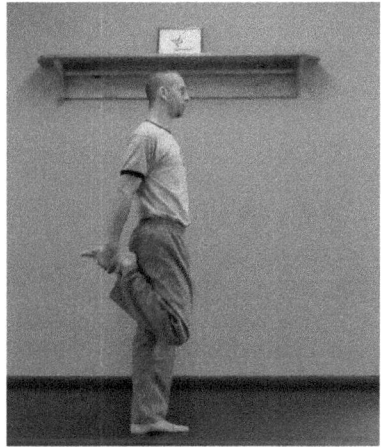

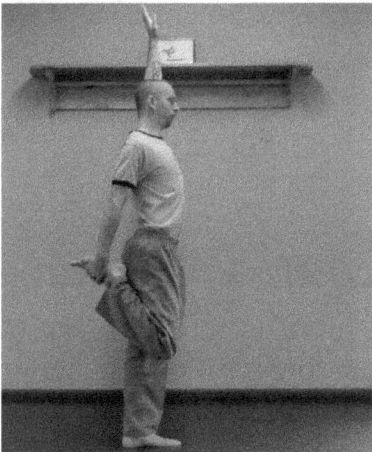

2. Raise the opposite hand toward the ceiling. Take a moment to maintain your balance. Focus your eyes straight ahead.

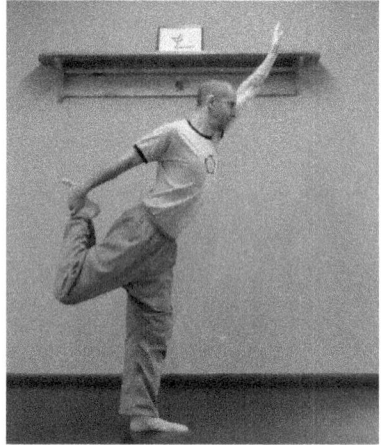

3. Bend forward at the waist, keeping the foot pulled upward in order to stretch the top of the thigh.

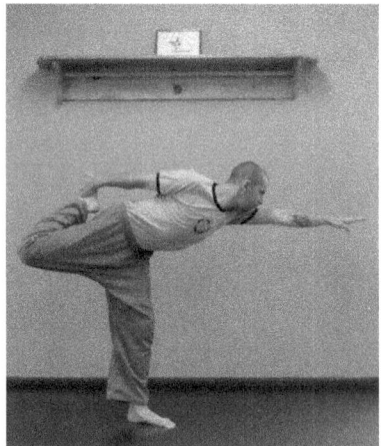

4. Continue bending forward Until the upper body and the thigh are parallel to the ground.

5. Slowly straighten up into a standing position. The more slowly you do the exercise, the more it will benefit you.

Dragon Roll

This is an old Taoist exercise. It massages the back muscles and the Taoists believed the massaging promoted health in the kidneys. In addition to the health aspects, it develops coordination useful in training practical applications of Pai Lum.

Sit with the feet in front of you a comfortable space apart.

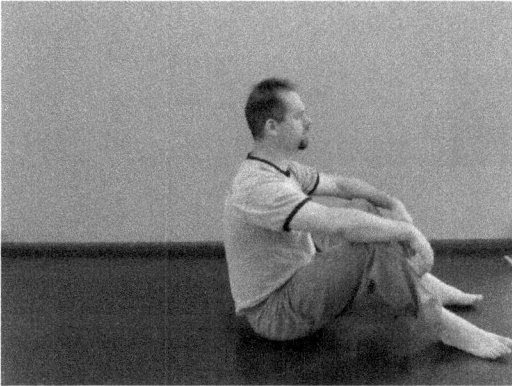

Keeping your weight off to the right side, roll backwards, keeping the chin tucked to avoid hitting back of the head.

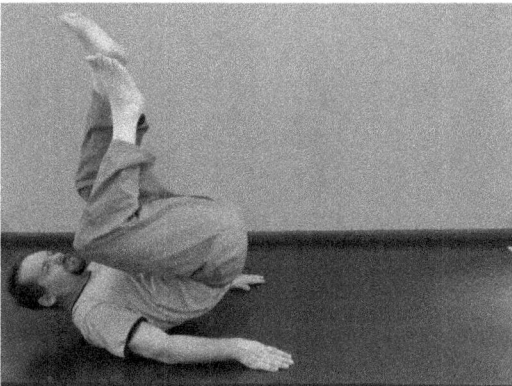

Forest Dragon Exercises

After rolling all the way back allow yourself to roll forward returning to the starting position. Repeat to the opposite side, along the left side of the back. Care should be taken to avoid

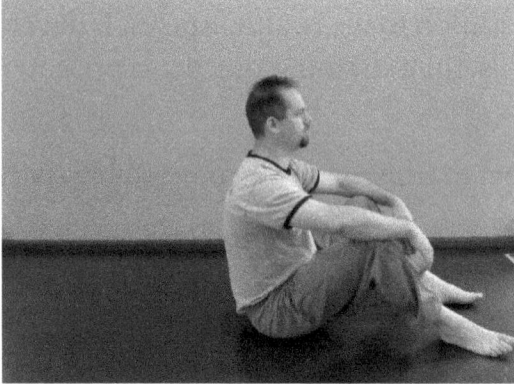

rolling along the spine. The contact with the ground goes from just above the right hip, along the right side of the back, and to the back of the right shoulder and then back along the side of the back to the hip as shown below, likewise on the left side as shown in the picture on the right.

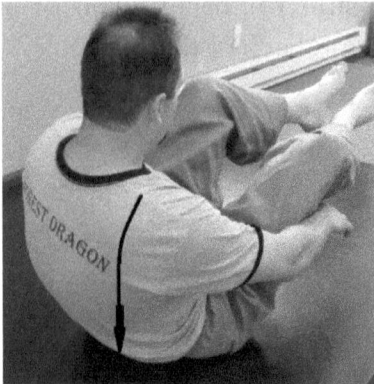

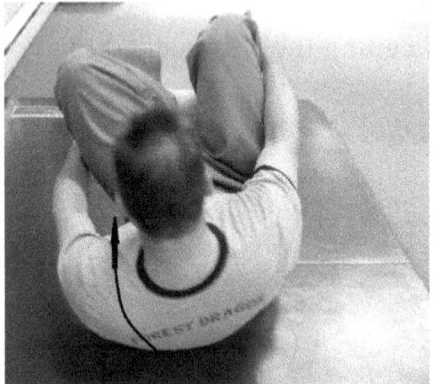

Do this 5 to 10 times on each side. On some days I find it helps to do more repetitions to loosen up the back muscles.

Head to Knee   (Paschimottanasana)

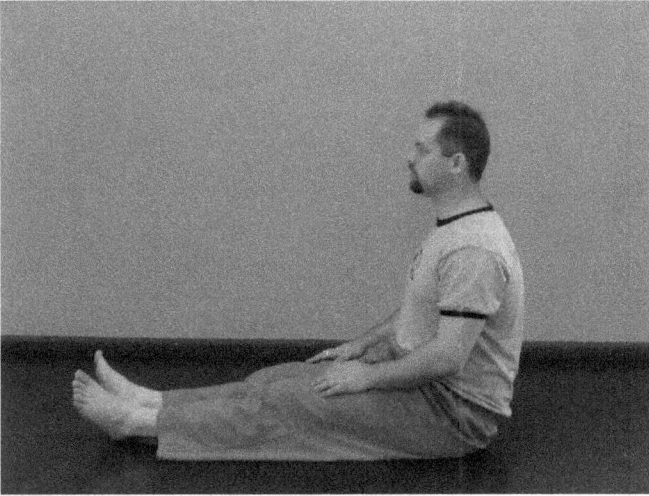

Begin by sitting on the floor with the legs together. Bend
forward placing the hands behind the knees. Relax and let
your weight pull your upper body toward your legs.

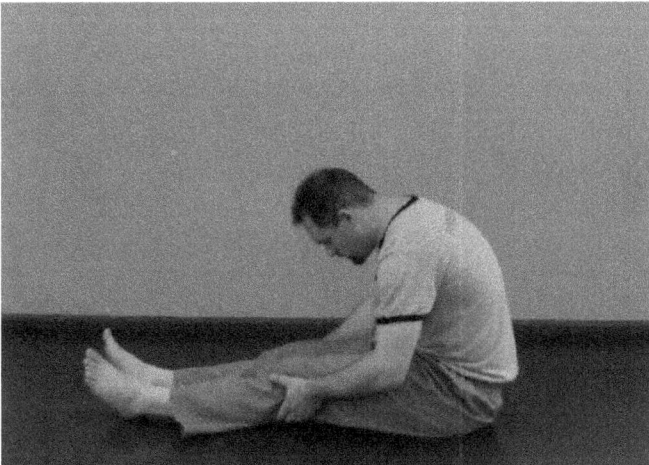

Forest Dragon Exercises

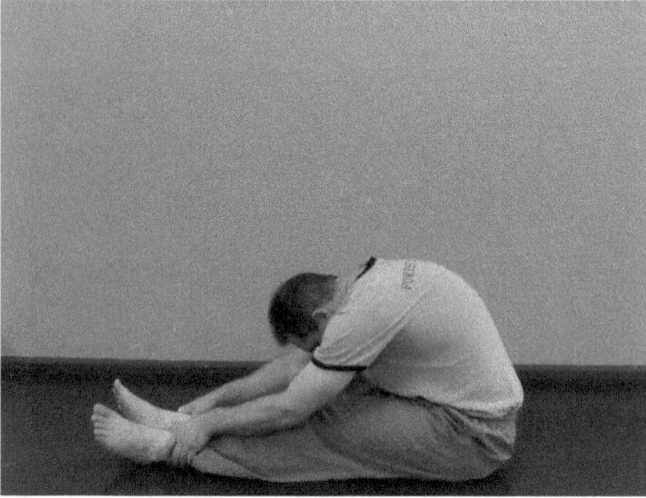

Gently pull your body towards your legs by grasping the back of the calves or the ankles. Allow the spine and neck to relax. You can then stretch the calf muscles by pulling the toes back toward you as shown below.

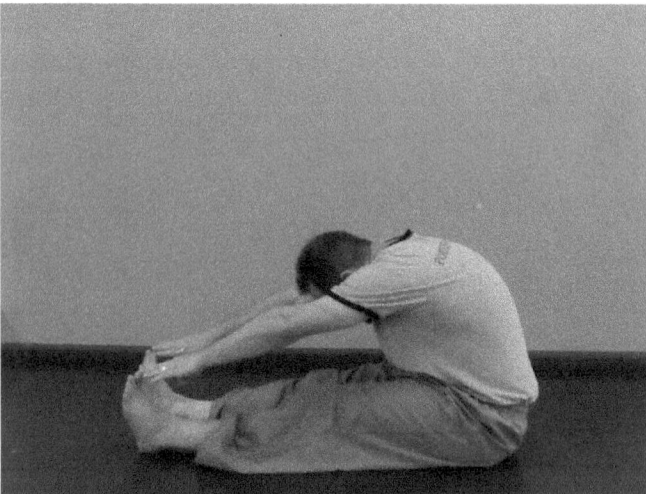

(Optional) As a variation, or in preparation for the head to knee exercise, the standing head to knee stretch can be done. This is known as *Uttanasana*.

Dragon Boat   (*Navasana*)

This exercise is essentially the same as the yoga posture *navasana*, which literally means "boat pose," although it is a simplified version of it. It is used to strengthen the abdominal muscles as well as the hip flexors. It also may aid digestion.

Begin by lying flat on your back.

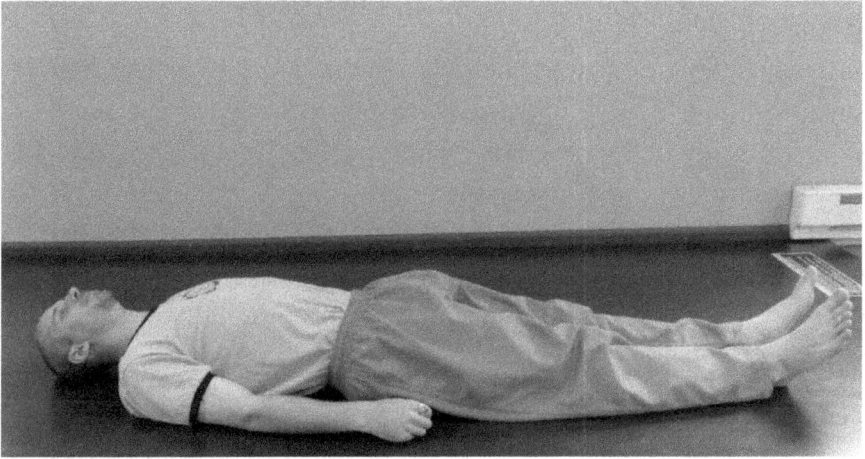

Simultaneously raise your chest and legs off of the floor, slowly of course.

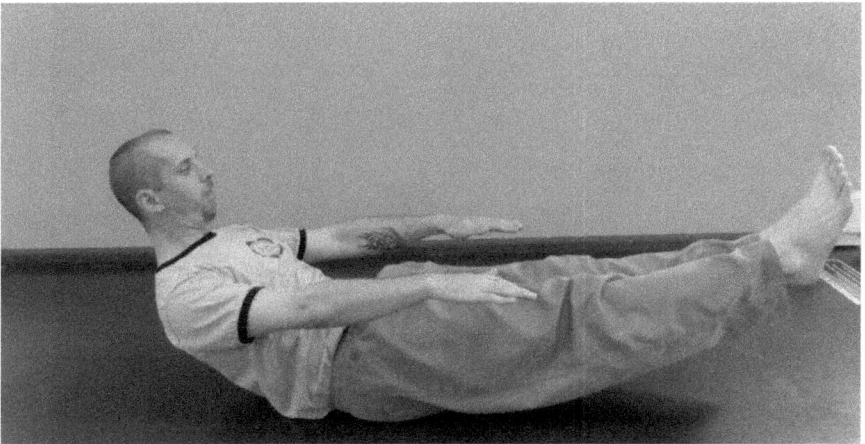

Continue bringing the upper body and legs up as far as you can while keeping the arms parallel to the ground. Continue to breathe naturally.

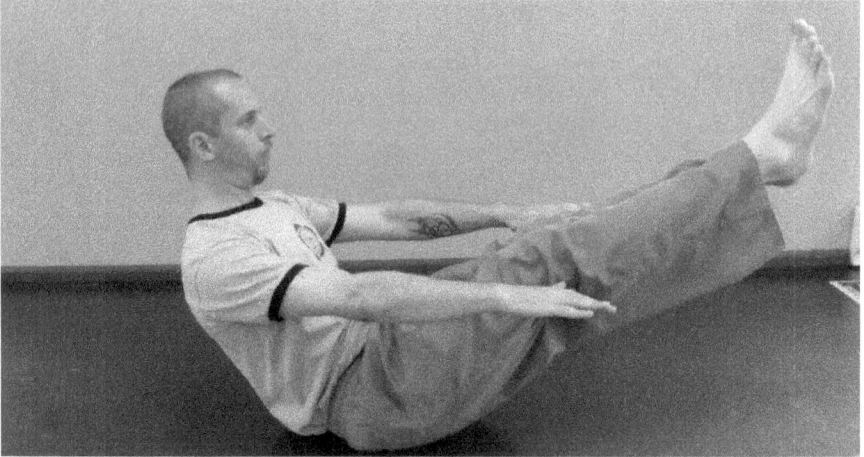

Slowly return to the starting position, trying your best to control your body's defiance of gravity. The more slowly you lower yourself, the more benefit you get from the exercise.

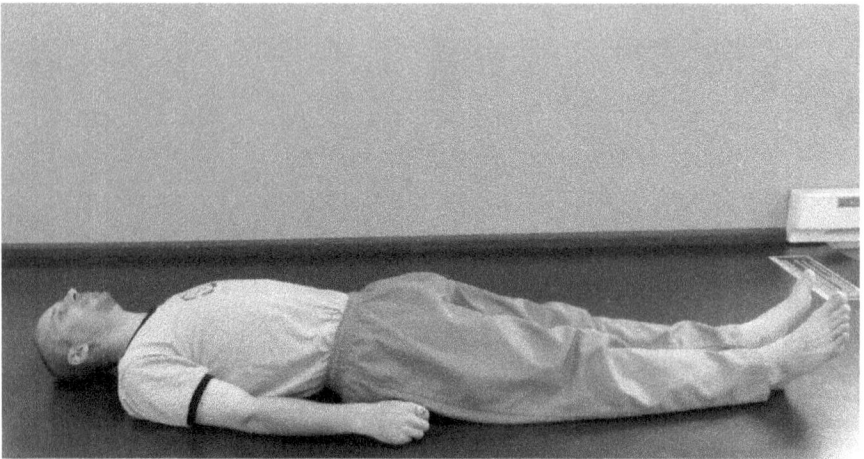

Forest Dragon Exercises

Movement Form
套路 (tao lu)

"In karate,

there is no advantage in the first attack."

- Gichin Funakoshi, Founder, Shotokan

The formal exercises or movement forms, known in Chinese as *tao lu*, provide a sequence of movements that are meant to develop coordination and balance as well as flexibility and stamina. At the same time, these movements provide the basics of the defense aspect of Forest Dragon exercises. They are performed as if the student were actually fighting, sometimes several opponents at once. For this reason they are sometimes referred to as fighting forms. These forms are a way of practicing techniques in a practical and less boring manner than simply simple repetitions of basic techniques.

There are five Forest Dragon forms, one for each of the five phases. They reflect the nature of each of the five elements and are designed to convey different concepts as the student progresses through the five phases of development.

This book does not go into detail on basic techniques such as a proper stance or how to form a proper fist. I chose to omit this level of detail for two reasons. For those only interested in the health benefits of the exercise these things are not that important. For those interested in the combative aspects of the art, I did not feel that these could be addressed properly in this brief training manual and highly recommend to the student that they find a good teacher to work with on proper technique, fighting concepts, and applications.

Many beginning students only view the forms as a set of techniques that can be used in application of "real world" situation. They are that indeed – but they are much more.

Forest Dragon Exercises

Each technique in a form is an example of a concept and how that concept can be applied in a specific situation. For example, a move in a form might be to step backward and block and then shift the weight forward and throwing a punch. This is a very simple technique that can be used to effectively defend against a front kick. But the real benefit is training the mind and body to evade an attack and then counterattack by moving the body effectively. The exact block and counter used with this concept can be varied to adapt to specific situations in many ways. Students are encouraged to be mindful of the movements and to let their minds explore the possibilities. That's what keeps it interesting.

The following conventions are used in the descriptions of the movements in their direction and orientation. The directions *north, south, east,* and *west* are used to describe direction or orientation relative to your surroundings. For example, if you are facing the front of a room when you begin, the front of the room represents *north,* the back of the room represents *south, east* is towards your right, and *west* is towards your left. These directions, like the walls of the room, remain the same from the beginning to the end of the exercise.

The directions *left, right, front,* and *back* are used to describe the direction of movement relative to your own body, specifically your hips. For example, if you are facing *north, left* will be towards the *west* wall; however, if you turn towards the *south, left* will be towards the *east* wall.

All forms begin and end with a bow. The bow in Chinese styles, also known as a salutation, is often complex compared to the typical bow used in Japanese schools and varies from one school to another.

For the sake of simplicity this book will use a "courtesy bow." This is simply making a fist with the right hand and covering it with the left hand. If you are training with an instructor, they will give you a specific way of executing the full formal salutation.

Young Dragon   *Earth*

Young Dragon introduces the student to some of the basic concepts of Pai Lum including commonly used stances, basic blocking techniques, several hand strikes, and the front kick. Movement is fairly simple, primarily forward and backward, side to side, and focuses on a single opponent in any given sequence of techniques.

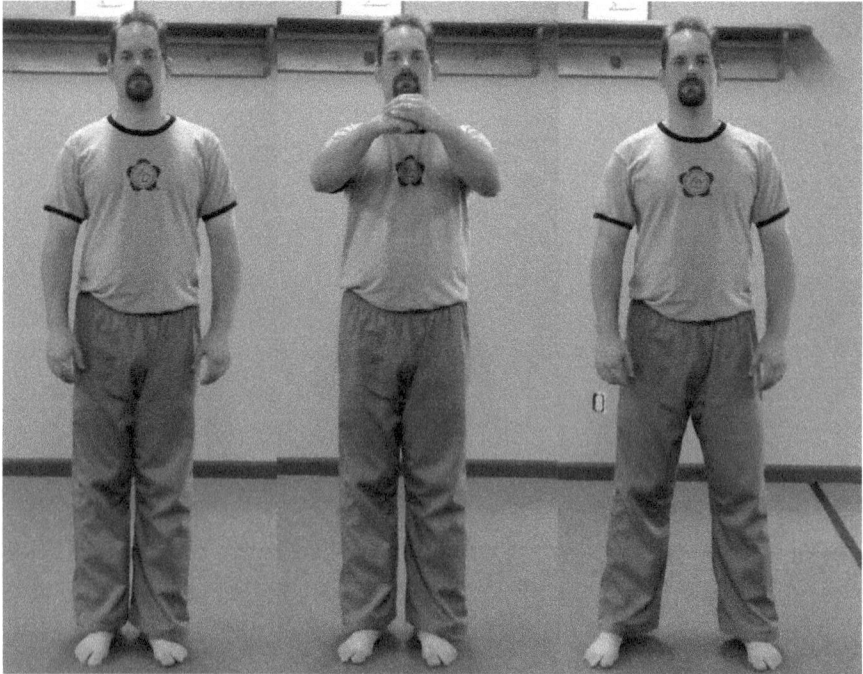

Begin with the hands at your sides and the feet together in attention stance. Perform a courtesy bow. Move the left foot to the left into a natural stance. The feet should be approximately shoulder width apart.

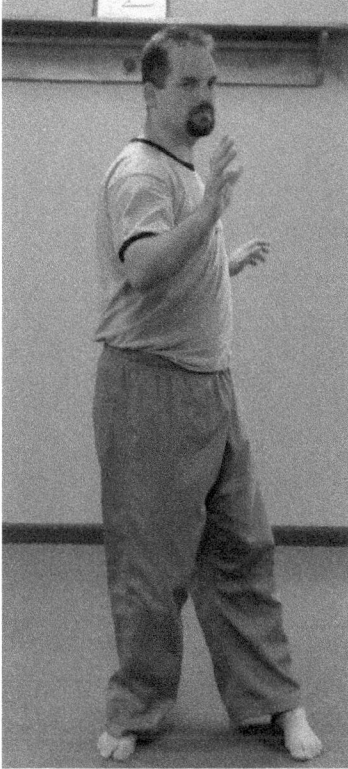

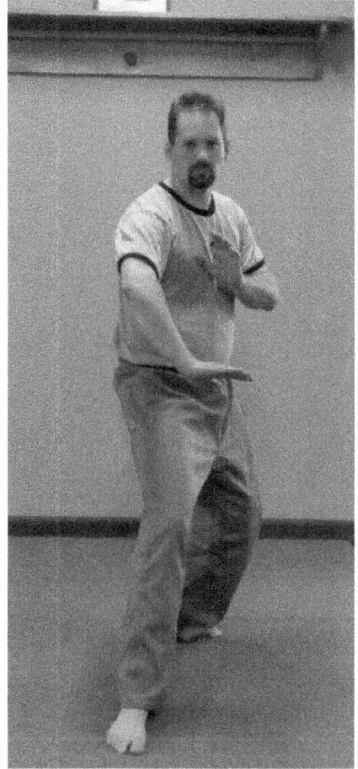

1. Shift weight over right foot as you turn hips to the left. The right hand rises north to face level slapping toward the left. Left foot steps to rear into right back stance; right hand continues circling counter-clockwise in lower level block, left hand pulls back into fist in guard position in front of solar plexus.

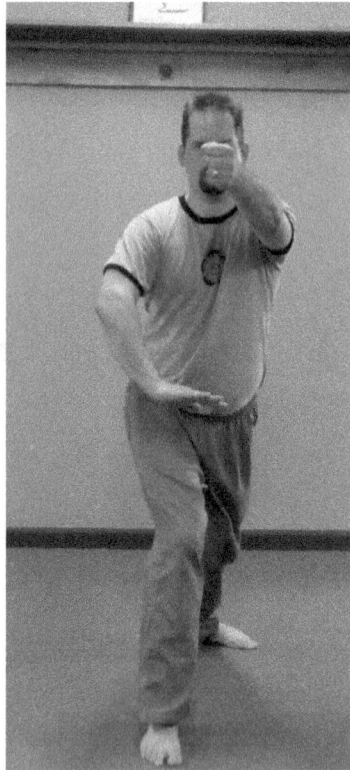

2. Extend forward into right forward stance; left vertical punch to face, right hand guards along centerline.

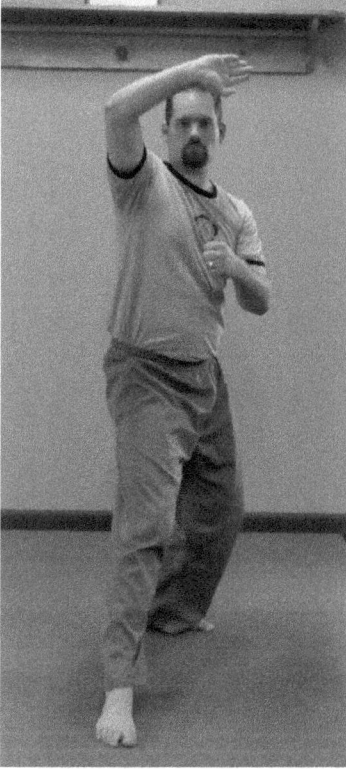

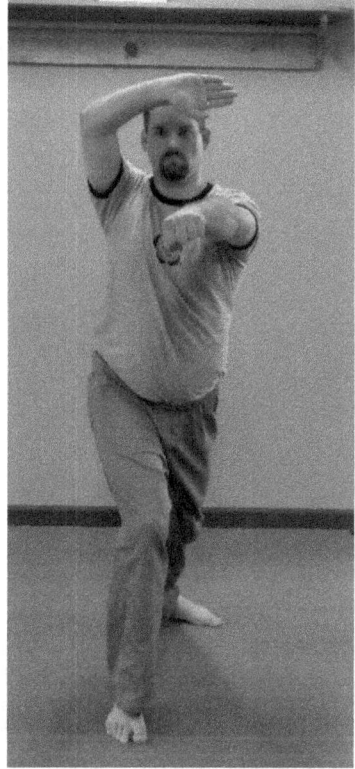

3. Shift weight back into right back stance; right hand executes upper area block, left hand pulls back into fist in guard position in front of solar plexus.

4. Extend forward into right forward stance; left straight punch to solar plexus, right hand guards head, fingers pointing towards left.

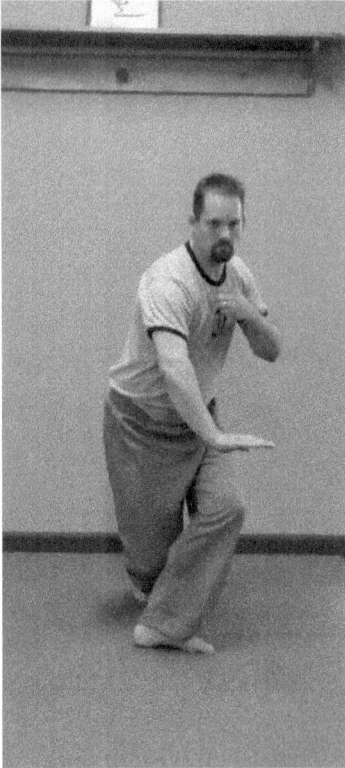

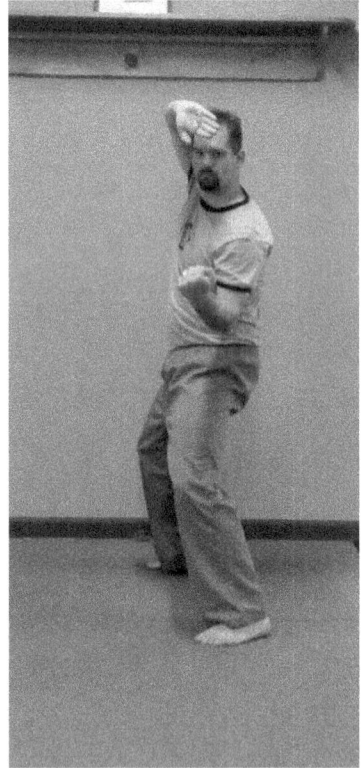

5. Right foot steps to rear into left monkey stance; right hand drops down into lower knife hand block to shin, left hand pulls back into fist in guard position by right shoulder.

6. Pivot right into horse stance (E); left upset punch to ribs, right hand guards head, fingers pointing down and left.

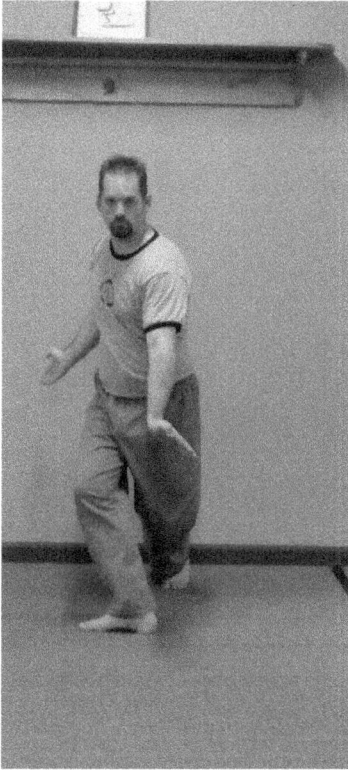

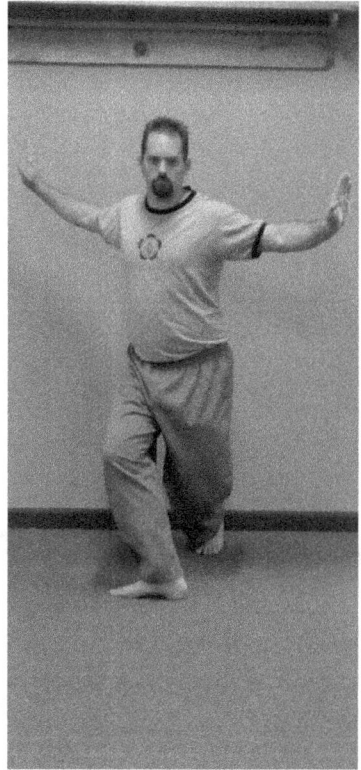

7. Left foot steps to rear into right monkey stance; left hand circles down into lower scooping block. Hands continue scooping movement, bringing hands upward.

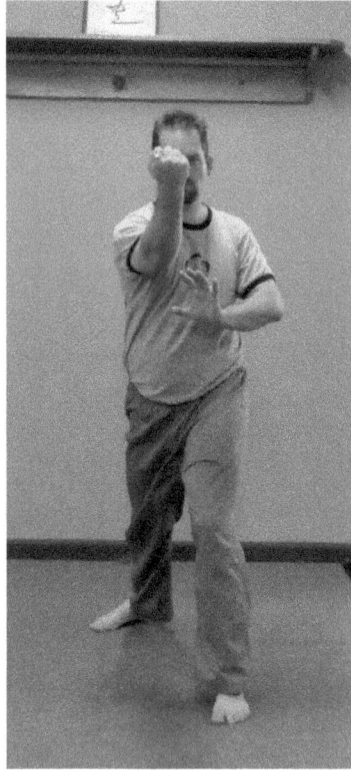

8. Left foot steps forward, extend into left forward stance; right hammer fist to temple, left hand guards along centerline, palm facing down.

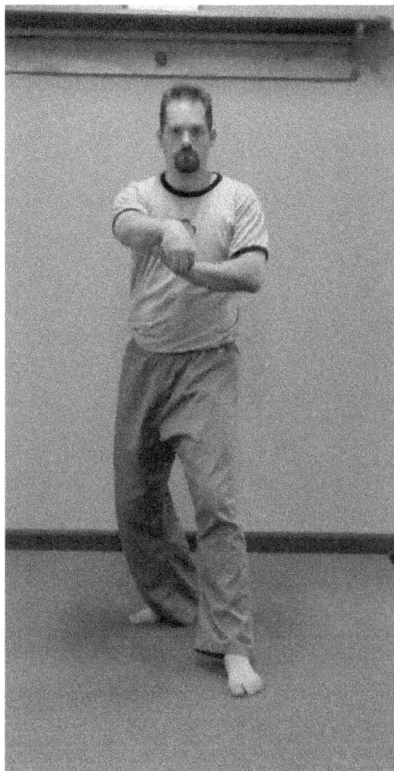

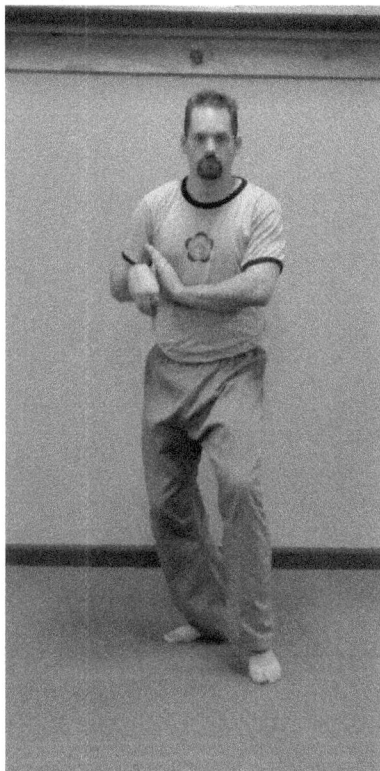

9. Right hand drops into hook, pull weight back over right foot in left cat stance; pull arms to the right in lower hooking block to side. Left hand at right wrist, fingers pointing upward (butterfly block).

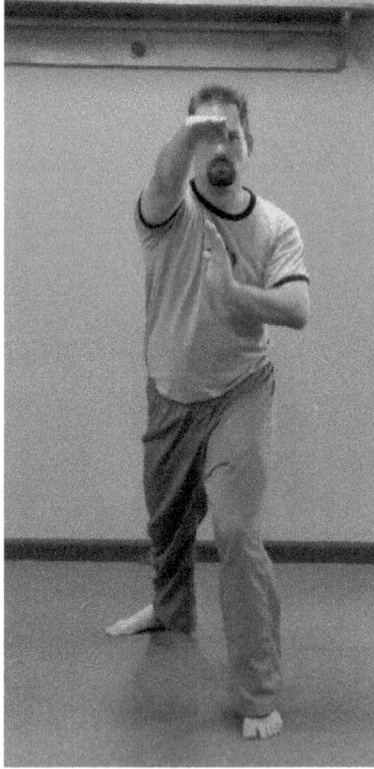

10. Step forward with left foot into left forward stance; bring right hand to temple in ridge hand strike, the left palm by forearm just below wrist.

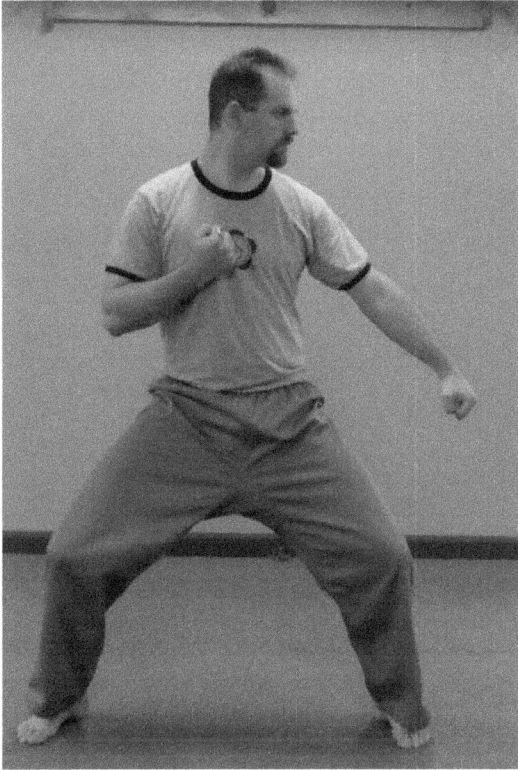

11. Right foot steps up into horse stance (N), left arm drops in forearm block to side, right hand in fist guarding just below left shoulder.

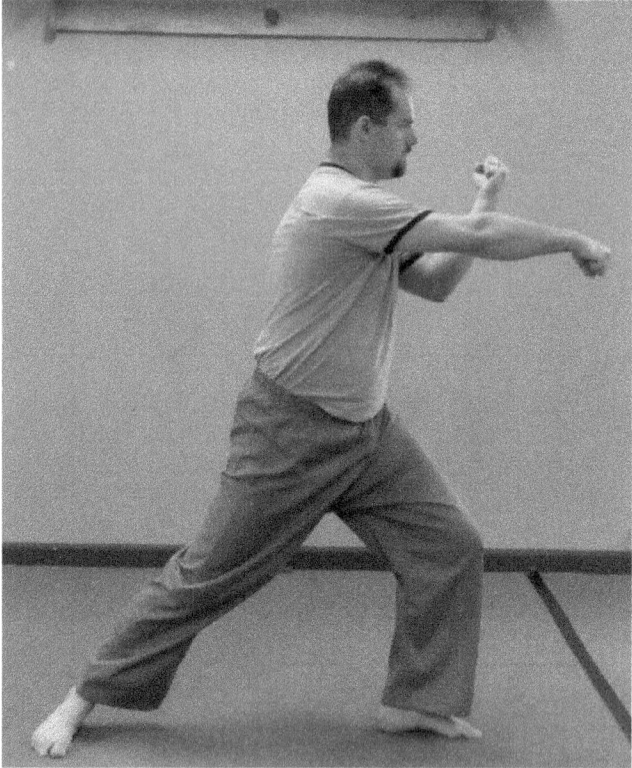

12. Pivot left into forward stance, right straight punch to left, left forearm guards along centerline.

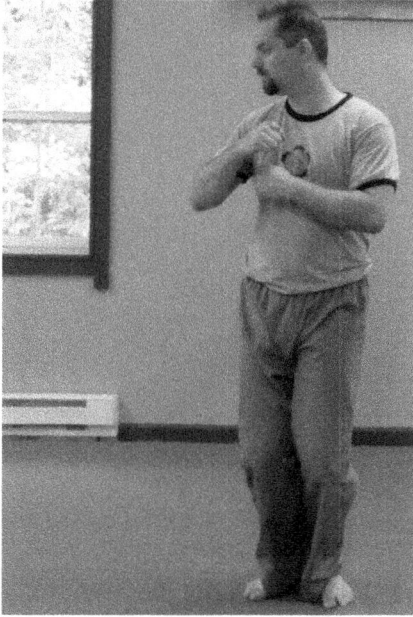

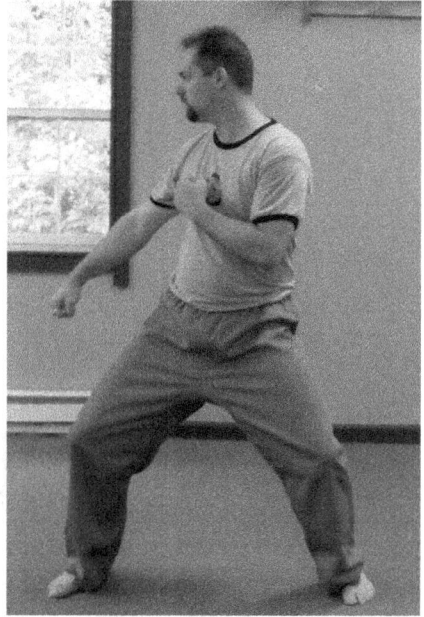

13. Pivot toward right bringing left foot up next to right foot.

Right arm drops in forearm block to side as right foot slides out into horse stance.

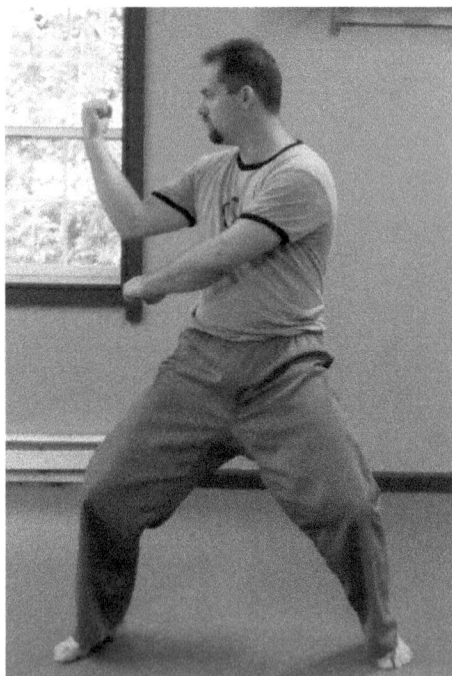

14. Left hook punch to right, right forearm guards along centerline.

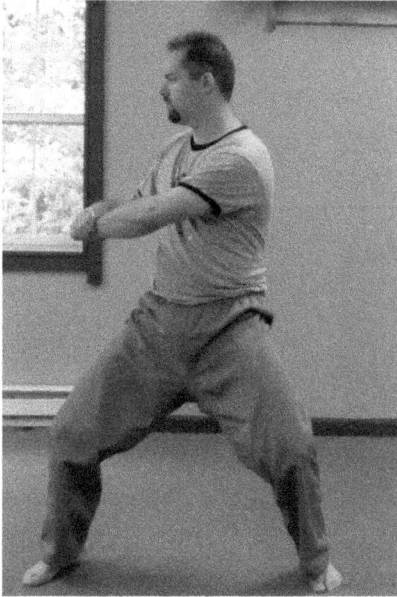

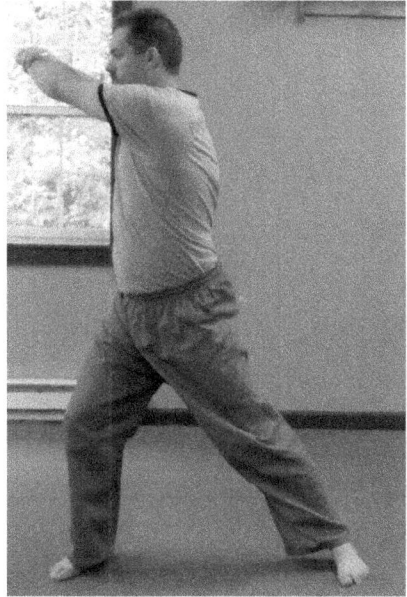

15. Right hand grabs top of left wrist, both hands immediately pull back to right side and rise upward…

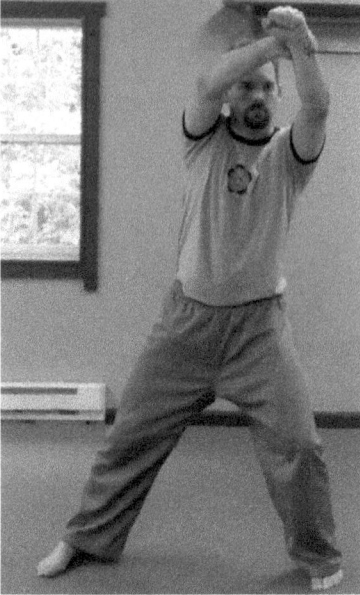

Left foot steps to NW as hands
continue counter-clockwise
overhead,

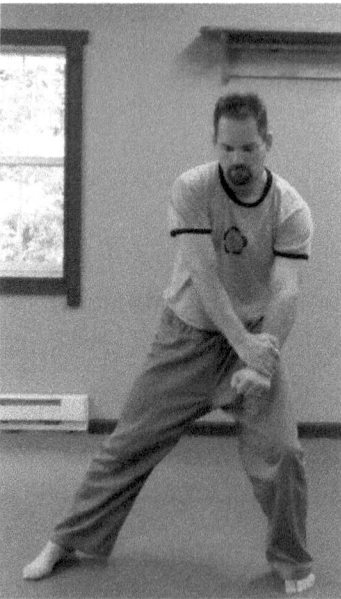

continue circling down alongside
left knee …

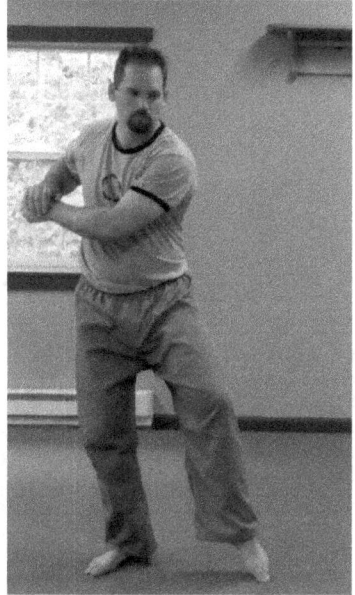

As hands continue circling, pull back into left cat stance, hands pull back by right hip.

16. Extend into left forward stance executing left palm heel downward inside left knee, right hand guards in front of centerline.

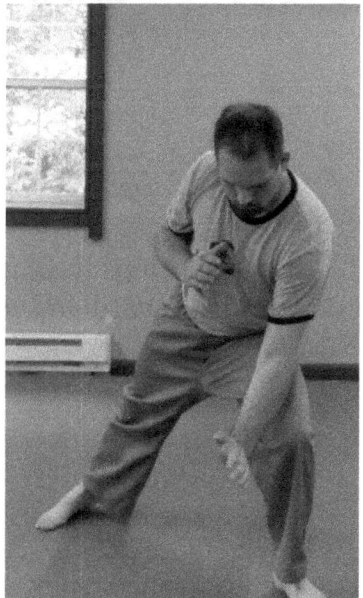

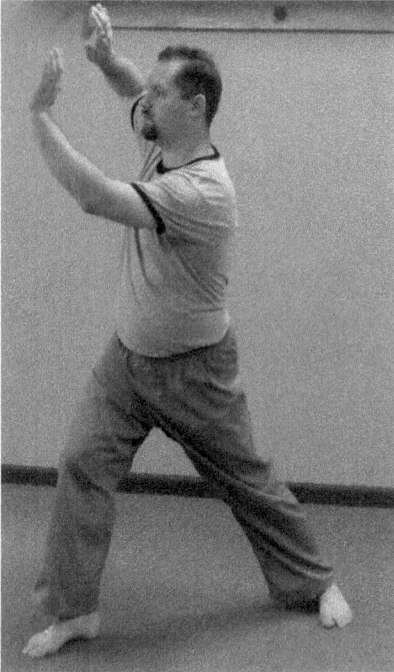

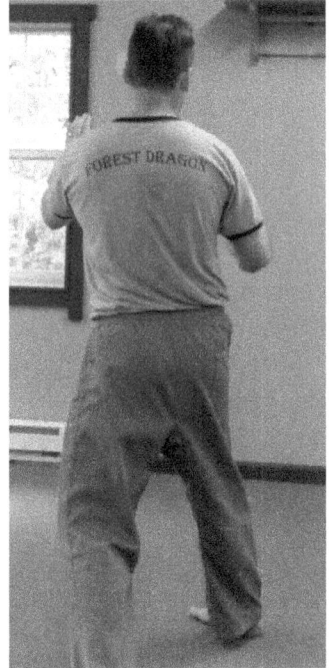

17. Right foot steps (NE) into forward stance while bringing both hands upward and to the right in double palm parry blocks. Continue moving on a diagonal (NE) with left foot followed by ...

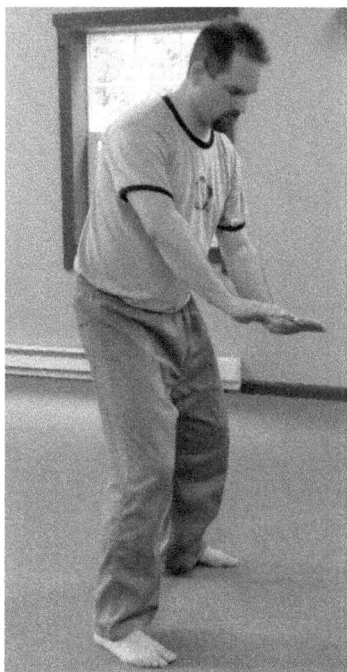

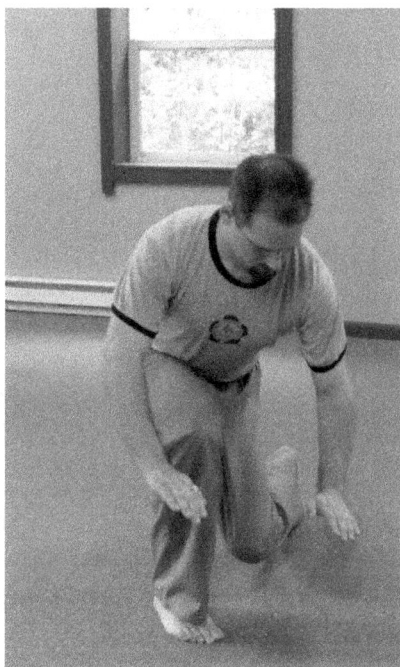

stepping with right foot behind and turning body to right 180°
and then bending left knee into left twisted stance facing (N).
Hands follow naturally in front of body and downward
executing takedown.

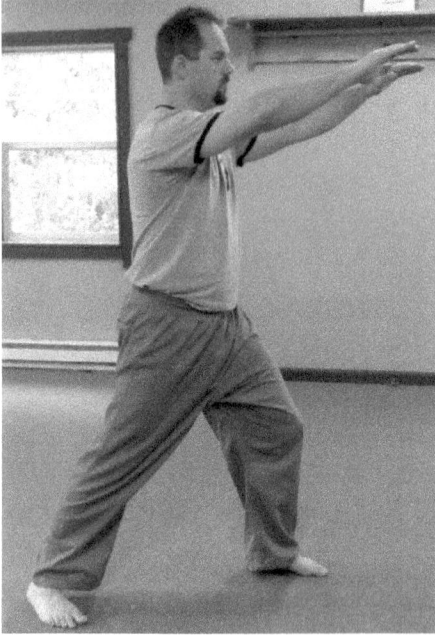

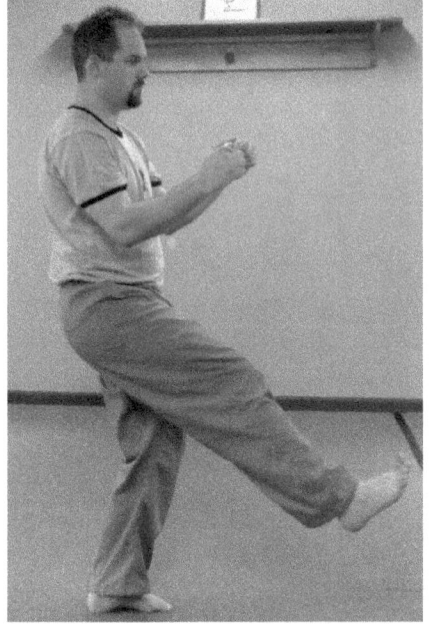

18. Left foot steps into left forward stance (W), hands extend in grab, execute right front kick to knee...

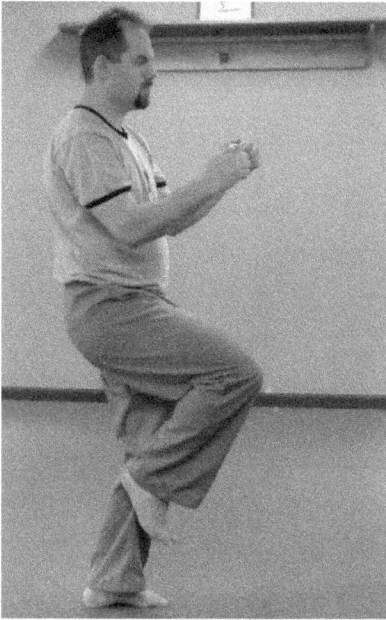

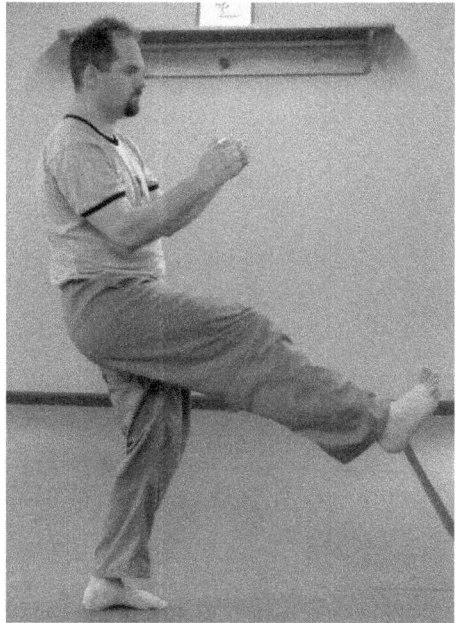

... followed by right front knife edge kick to groin.

Right foot steps down while turning into left forward stance (S), left hand extended in guard.

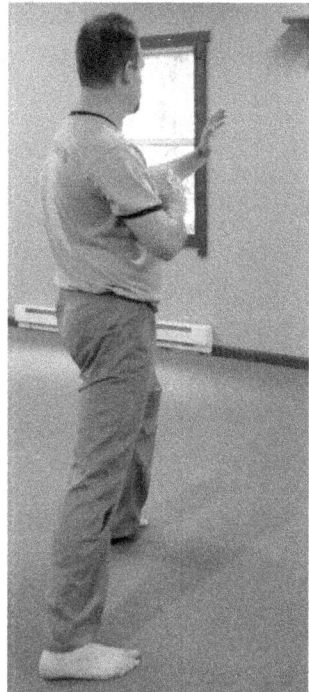

69

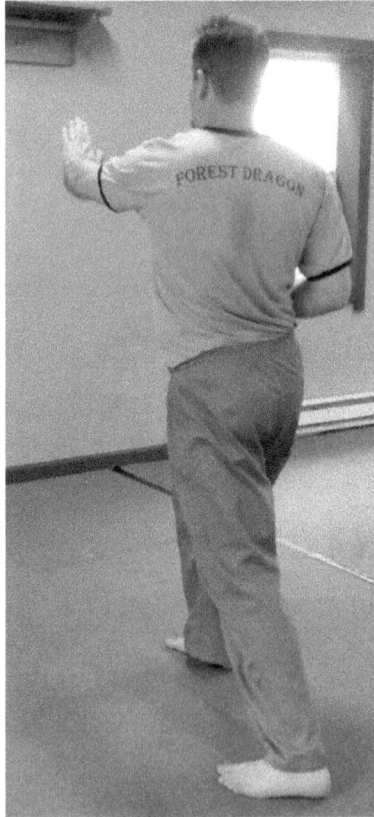

19. Right foot steps forward into right forward stance extending left palm heel in short strike to chest..

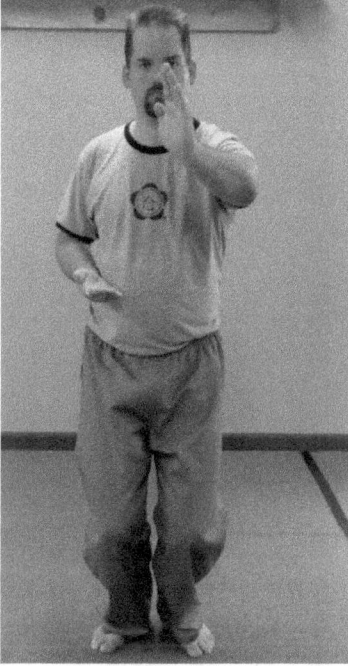
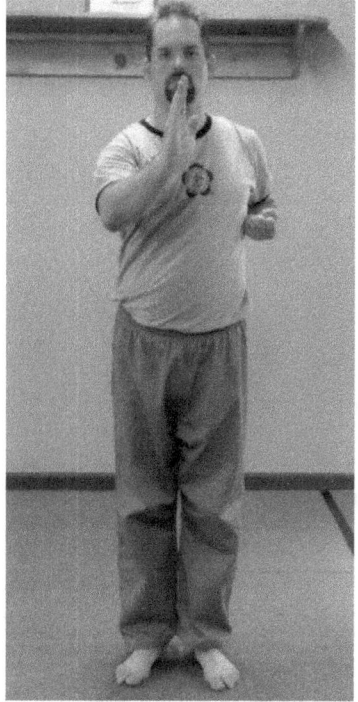

20. Turn 180° left while bringing left foot up next to right; straighten legs, rising into attention stance while extending right hand in willow leaf palm.

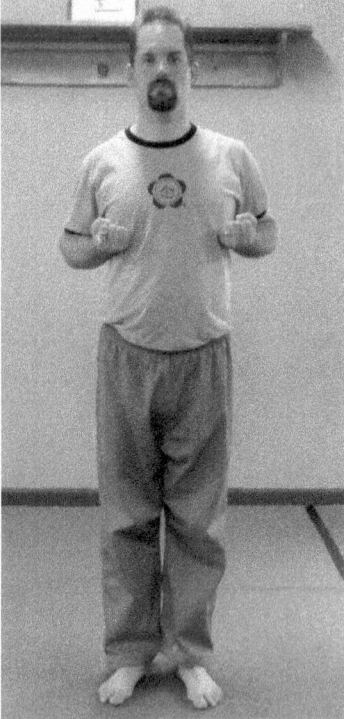

Pull left hand back in fist.

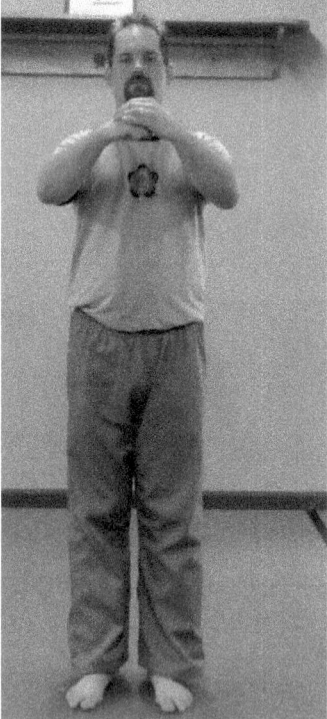

Finish by performing the bow.

Summary of Moves

1. Shift weight over right foot as you turn hips to the left. The right hand rises north to face level slapping toward the left. Left foot steps to rear into right back stance; right hand continues circling counter-clockwise in lower level block, left hand pulls back into fist in guard position in front of solar plexus.

2. Extend forward into right forward stance; left vertical punch to face, right hand guards along centerline.

3. Shift weight back into right back stance; right hand executes upper area block, left hand pulls back into fist in guard position in front of solar plexus.

4. Extend forward into right forward stance; left straight punch to solar plexus, right hand guards head, fingers pointing towards left.

5. Right foot steps to rear into left monkey stance; right hand drops down into lower knife hand block to shin, left hand pulls back into fist in guard position by right shoulder.

6. Pivot right into horse stance (E); left upset punch to ribs, right hand guards head, fingers pointing down and left.

7. Left foot steps to rear into right monkey stance; left hand circles down into lower scooping block. Hands continue scooping movement, bringing hands upward.

8. Left foot steps forward, extend into left forward stance; right hammer fist to temple, left hand guards along centerline, palm facing down.

9. Right hand drops into hook, pull weight back over right foot in left cat stance; pull arms to the right in lower hooking block to side. Left hand at right wrist, fingers pointing upward (butterfly block).

10. Step forward with left foot into left forward stance; bring right hand to temple in ridge hand strike, the left palm by forearm just below wrist.

11. Right foot steps up into horse stance (N), left arm drops in forearm block to side, right hand in fist guarding just below left shoulder.

12. Pivot left into forward stance, right straight punch to left, left forearm guards along centerline.

13. Pivot toward right bringing left foot up next to right foot. Right arm drops in forearm block to side as right foot slides out into horse stance.

14. Left hook punch to right, right forearm guards along centerline.

15. Right hand grabs top of left wrist, both hands immediately pull back to right side and rise upward. Left foot steps to NW in left forward and hands continue counter-clockwise overhead, continue circling down alongside left knee. As hands continue circling, pull back into left cat stance, hands pull back by right hip.

16. Extend into left forward stance executing left palm heel downward inside left knee, right hand guards in front of centerline.

17. Right foot steps (NE) into forward stance while bringing both hands upward and to the right in double palm parry blocks. Continue moving on a diagonal (NE) with left foot followed by stepping with right foot behind and turning body to right 180° and then bending left knee into left twisted stance facing (N). Hands follow naturally in front of body and downward executing takedown.

18. Left foot steps into left forward stance (W), hands extend in grab, execute right front kick to knee followed by right front knife edge kick to groin. Right foot steps down while turning into left forward stance (S), left hand extended in guard.

19. Right foot steps forward into right forward stance extending left palm heel in short strike to chest.

20. Turn 180° left while bringing left foot up next to right; straighten legs, rising into attention stance while extending right hand in willow leaf palm and pulling left hand back in fist.

Bow

Forest Dragon Exercises

Defense Applications

The movements of the Young Dragon form are meant to be effective as fighting techniques. Movements in martial arts forms and techniques can be applied to various situations in many different ways. This section demonstrates what I consider to be some of the simplest examples and should be considered a starting point for the student. Take these and practice them until they feel comfortable and natural. It is important that you are able to execute them with a training partner without having to think. As with other aspects of training it is important to remain mindful. When the mind and body are thoroughly familiar with the technique they will become integrated and work in unison. Only then will they be useful in a real situation.

Once you are comfortable with these examples, I encourage you to experiment with the movements and their application. This is some of the most challenging as well as the most rewarding part of practicing a martial art.

The techniques on the following pages are numbered in to make it easier for you to see which movements of the Young Dragon form are being demonstrated in application.

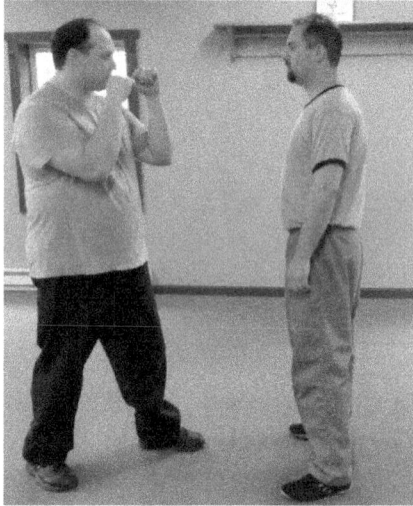

1. Shift weight over right foot as you turn hips to the left. The right hand rises north to face level slapping toward the left.

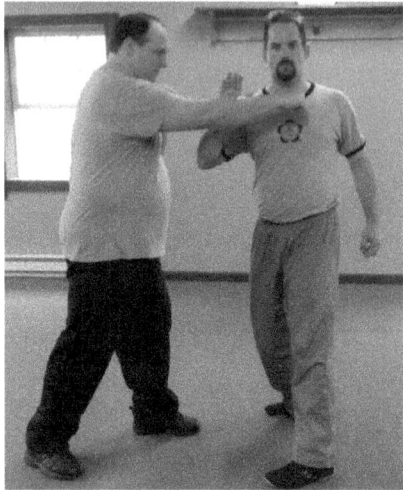

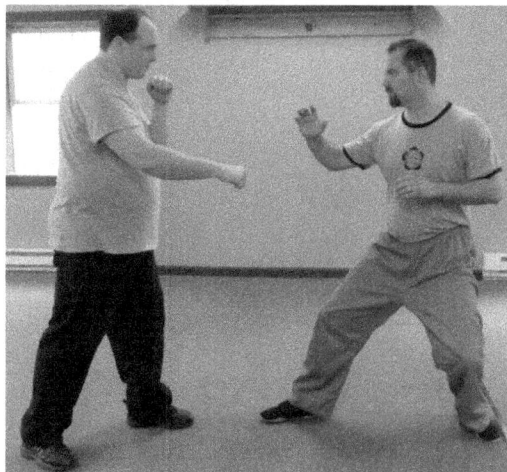

Left foot steps to rear into right back stance; right hand continues circling counter-clockwise in lower level block, left hand pulls back into fist in guard position in front of solar plexus.

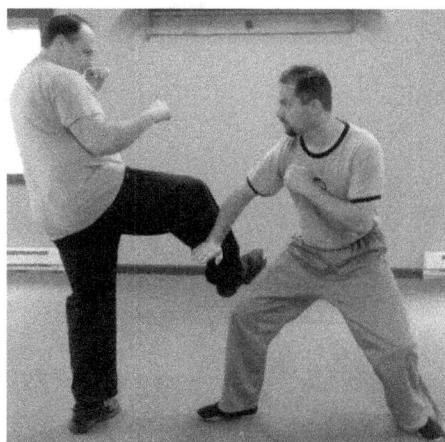

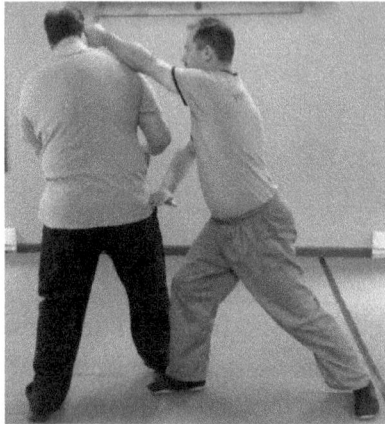

2. Extend forward into right forward stance; left vertical punch to face, right hand guards along centerline.

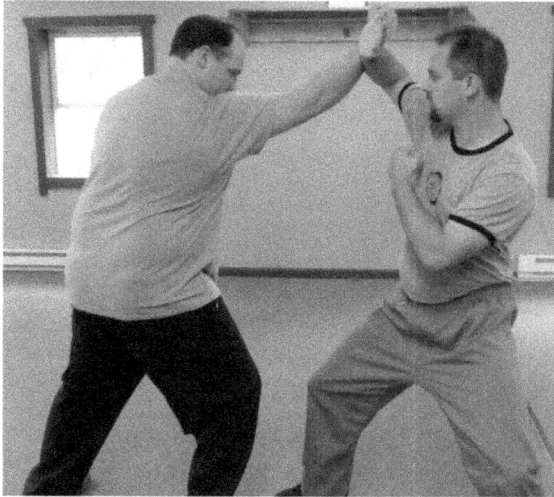

3. Shift weight back into right back stance; right hand executes upper area block, left hand pulls back into fist in guard position in front of solar plexus.

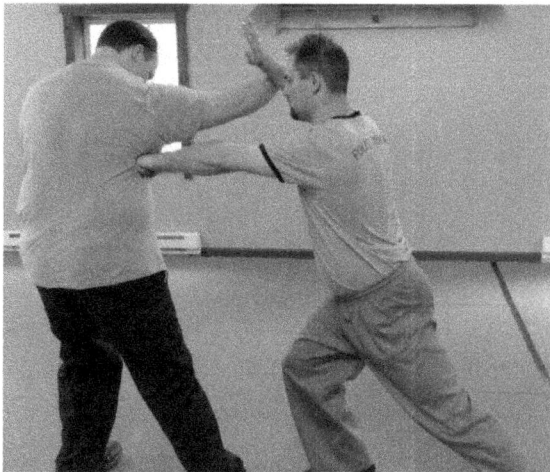

4. Extend forward into right forward stance; left straight punch to solar plexus, right hand guards head, fingers pointing towards left.

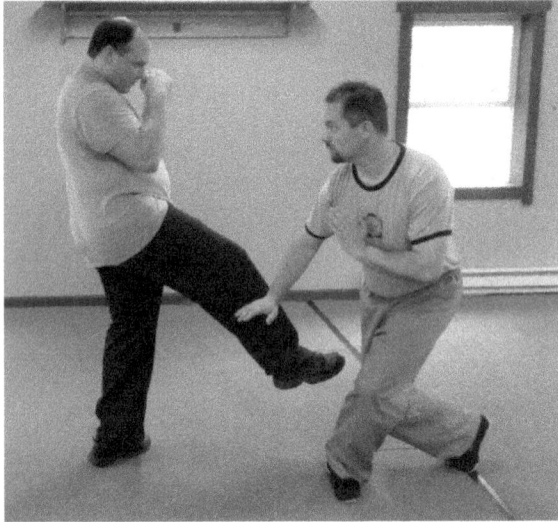

5. Right foot steps to rear into left monkey stance; right hand drops down into lower knife hand block to shin, left hand pulls back into fist in guard position by right shoulder.

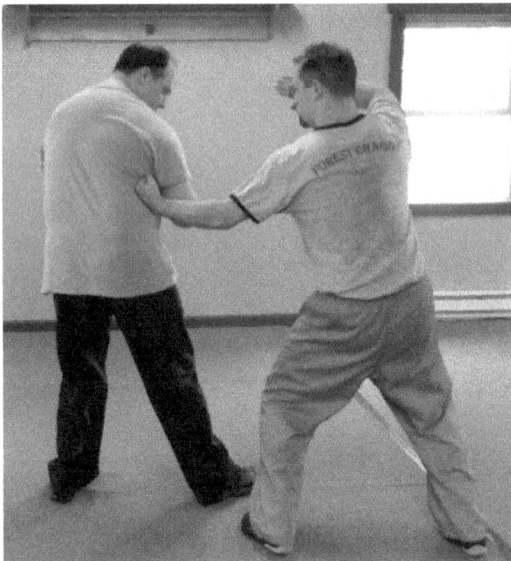

6. Pivot right into horse stance (E); left upset punch to ribs, right hand guards head, fingers pointing down and left.

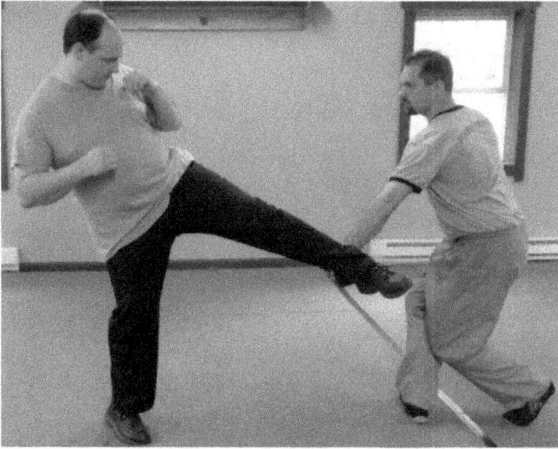

7. Left foot steps to rear into right monkey stance; left hand circles down into lower scooping block.

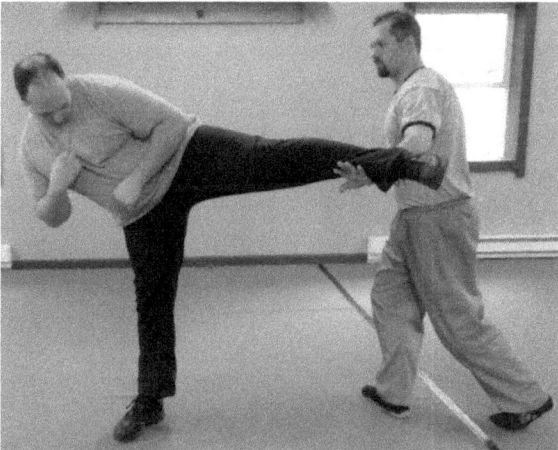

Hands continue scooping movement, bringing hands upward.

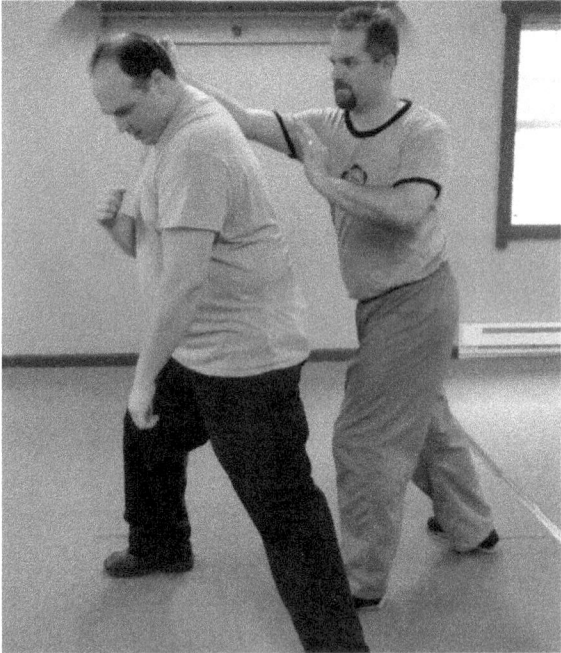

8. Left foot steps forward, extend into left forward stance; right hammer fist to temple, left hand guards along centerline, palm facing down.

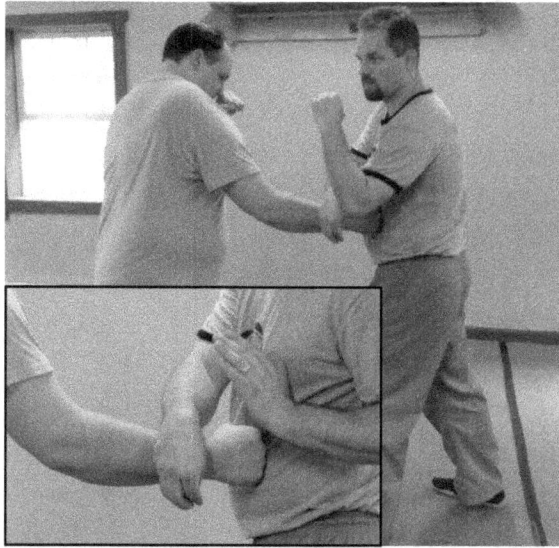

9. Right hand drops into hook, pull weight back over right foot in left cat stance; pull arms to the right in lower hooking block to side. Left hand at right wrist, fingers pointing upward (butterfly block).

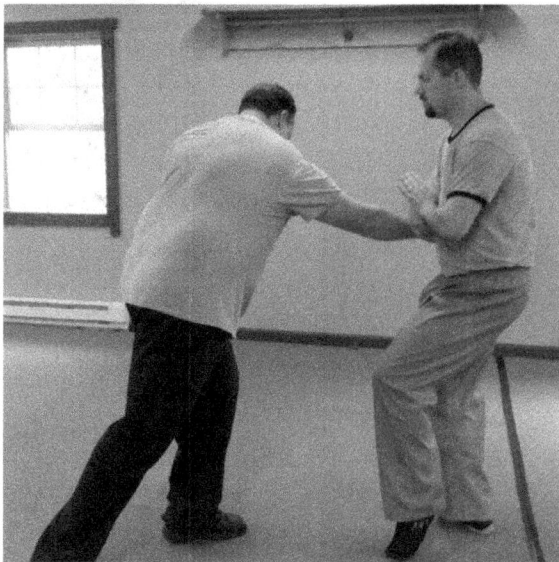

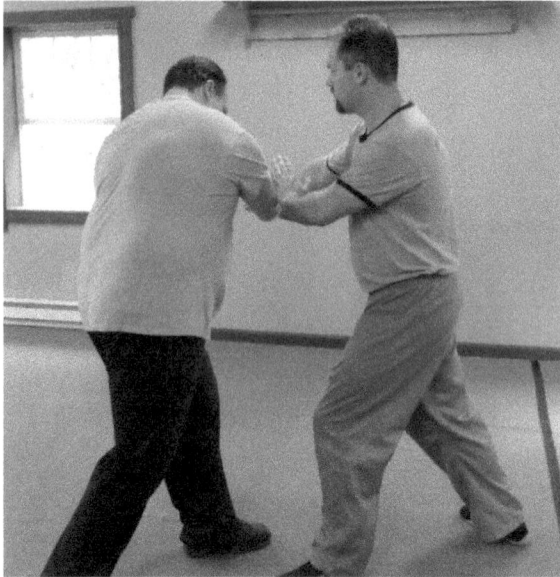

10. Step forward with left foot into left forward stance;

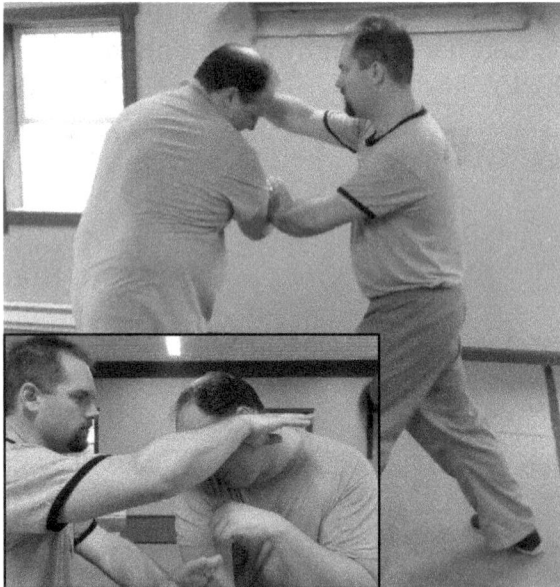

bring right hand to temple in ridge hand strike, the left palm by forearm just below wrist.

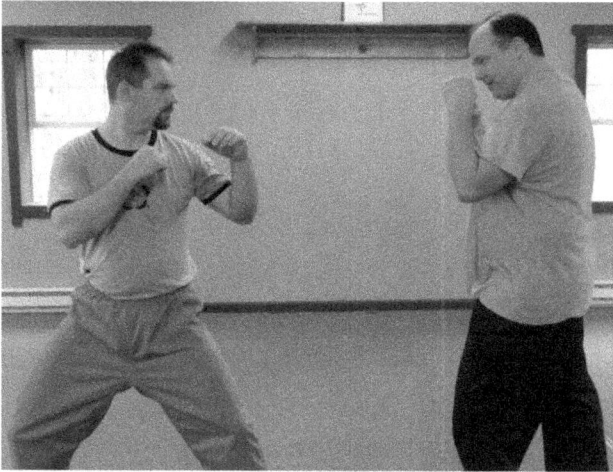

11. Right foot steps up into horse stance (N),

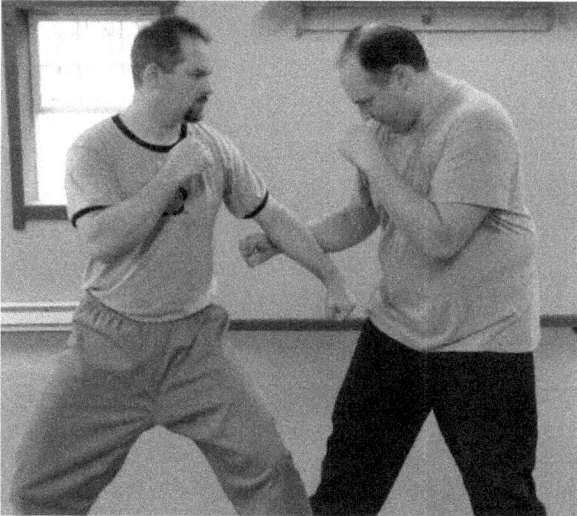

left arm drops in forearm block to side, right hand in fist guarding just below left shoulder.

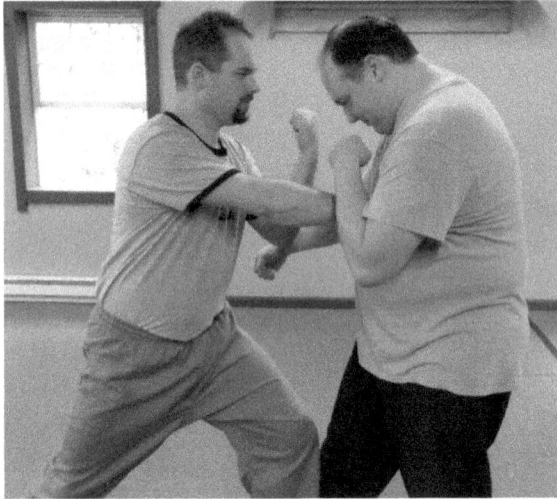

12. Pivot left into forward stance, right straight punch to left, left forearm guards along centerline.

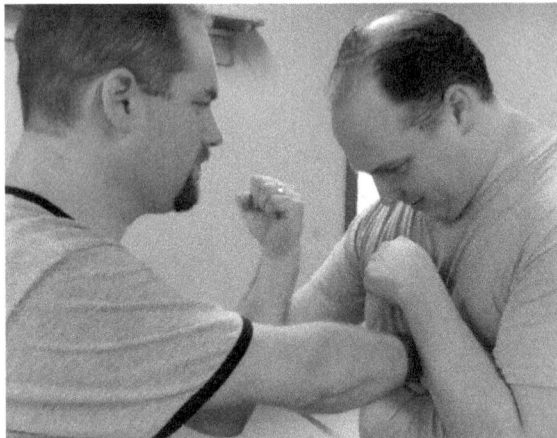

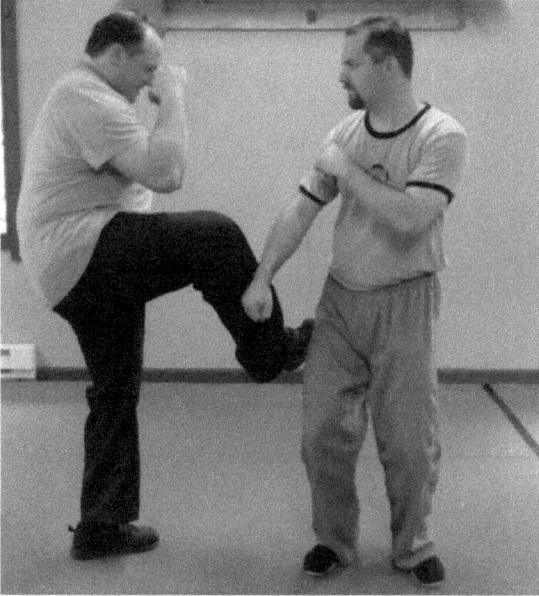

13. Pivot toward right bringing left foot up next to right foot. Right arm drops in forearm block to side as right foot begins slide into horse stance.

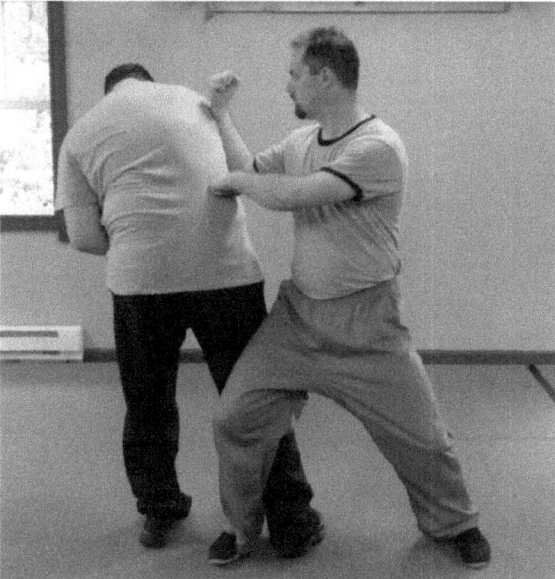

14. Left hook punch to right, right forearm guards along centerline.

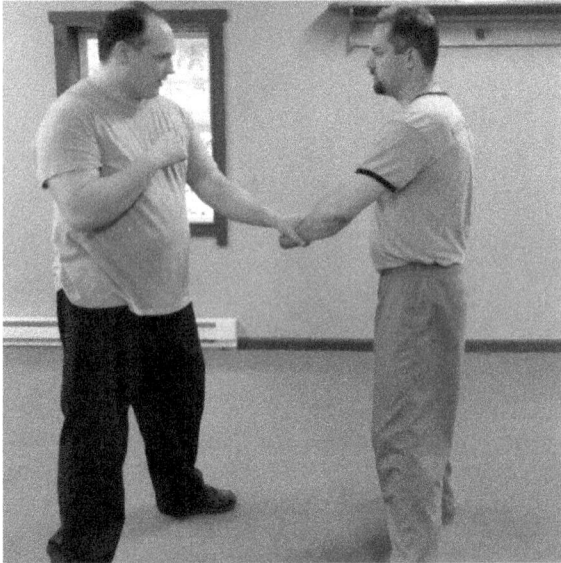

Opponent grabs your left wrist with his left hand.

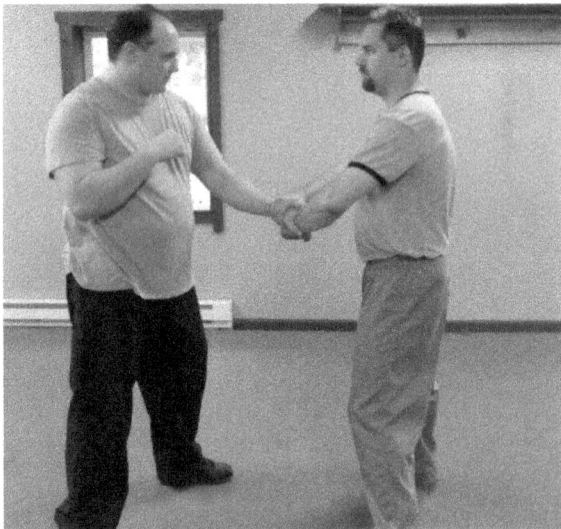

15. Right hand grabs top of left wrist,

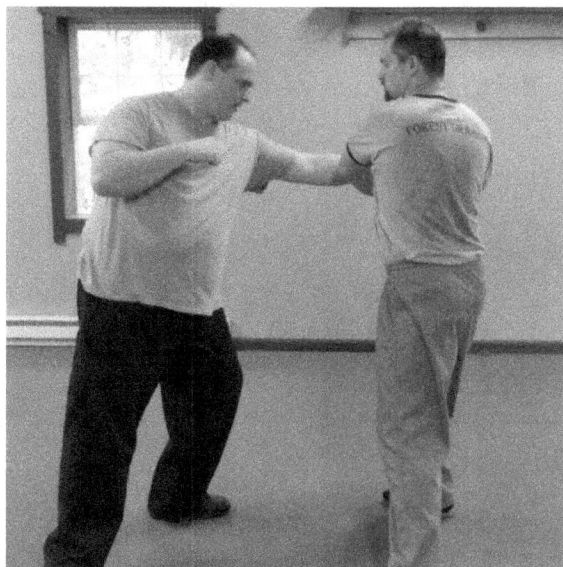

both hands pull back to right side and rise upward

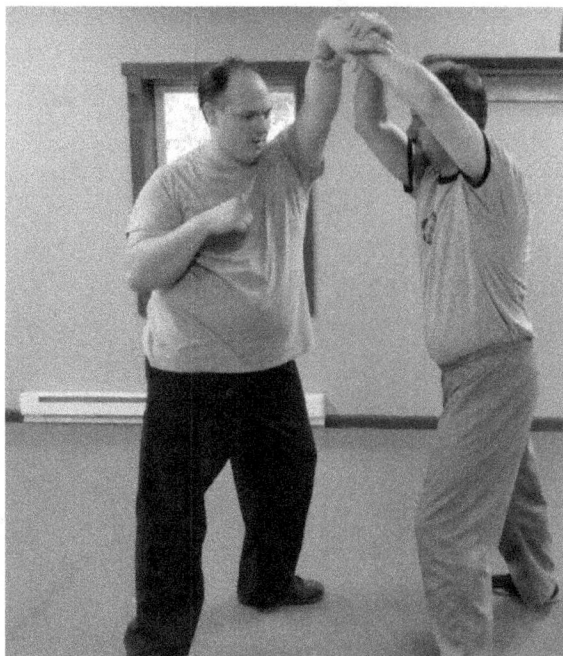

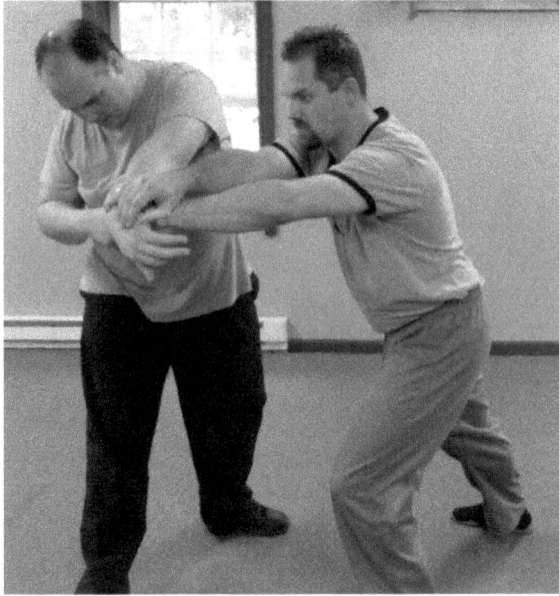

Left foot steps to NW in left forward and hands continue counter-clockwise overhead, continue circling down alongside left knee.

As hands continue circling, pull back into left cat stance, hands pull back by right hip (shown without opponent).

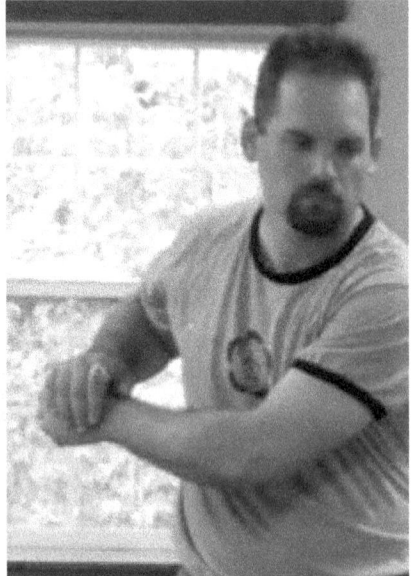

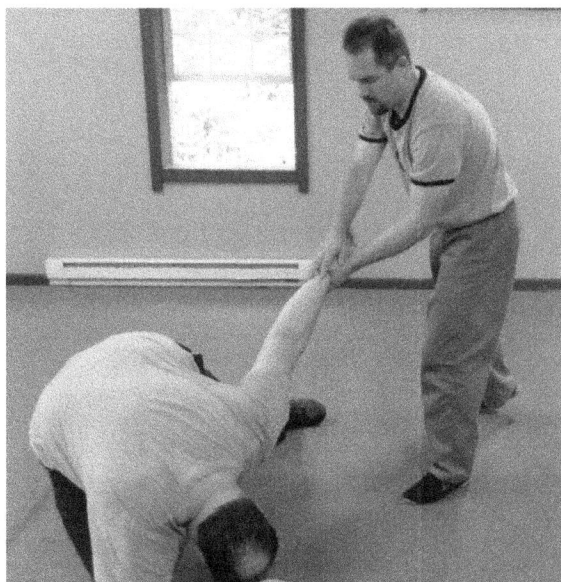

16. Extend into left forward stance executing left palm heel downward inside left knee, right hand guards in front of centerline. Bend right knee to get lower and closer to target.

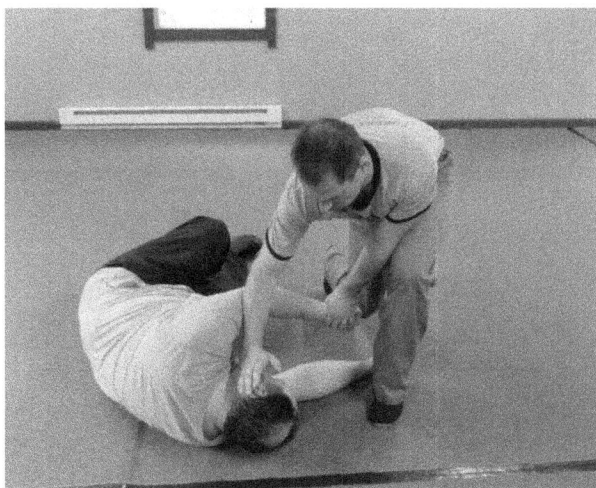

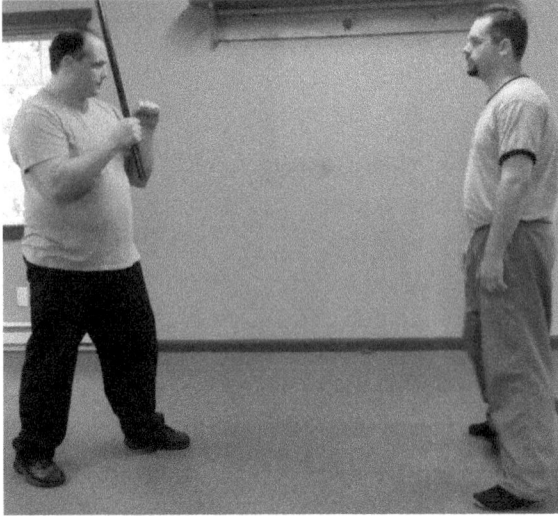

17. Attacker steps in with overhead strike toward head.

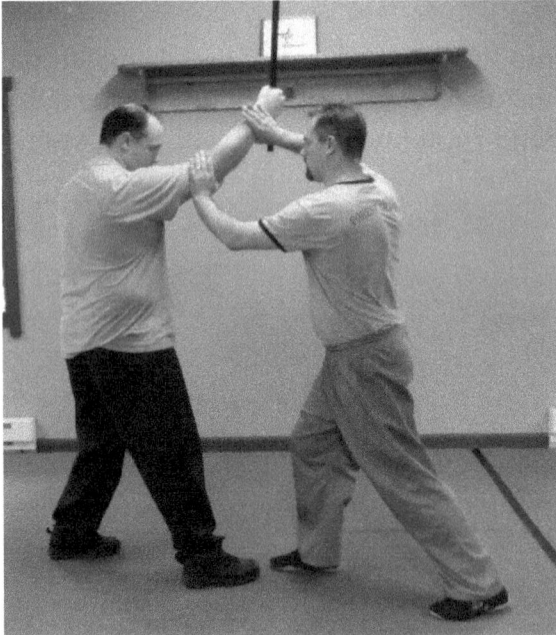

Right foot steps forward while bringing both hands
upward and to the right in double palm parry blocks.

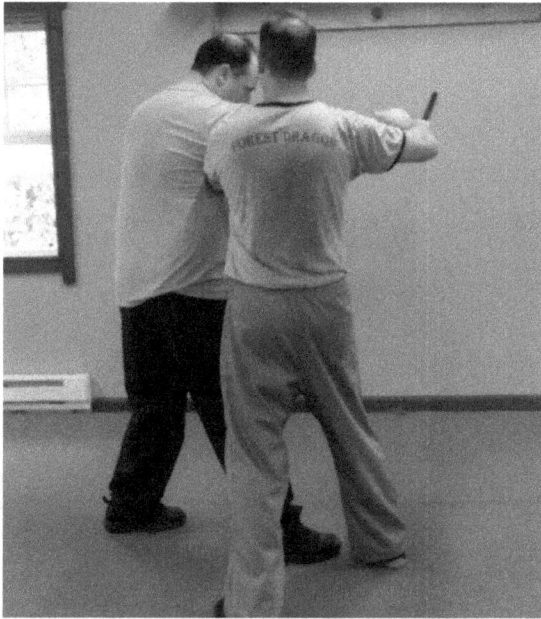

Continue moving on a diagonal (NE) stepping with left foot

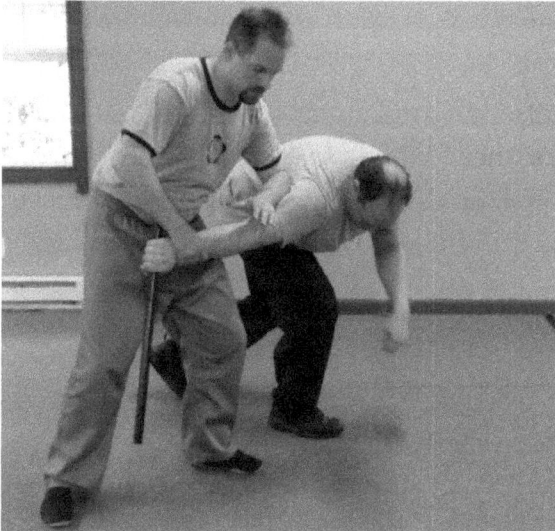

followed by stepping behind with right foot and turning body
to right 180°

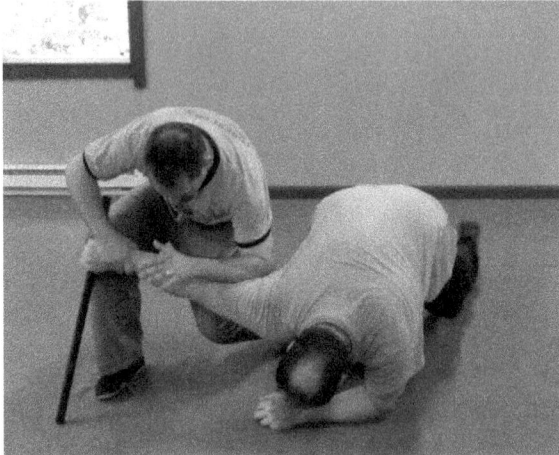

Continue motion by turning and bending left knee downward into twisted stance. Hands follow naturally in front of body and downward, holding wrist and applying pressure with left forearm, executing takedown.

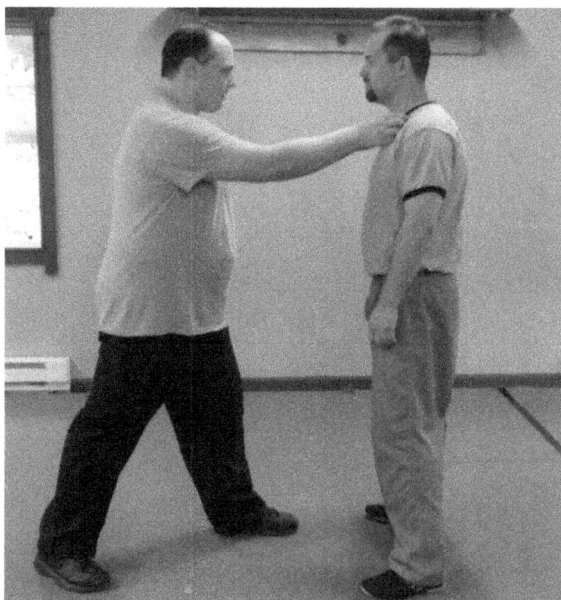

18. Opponent grabs shirt with both hands. Left foot steps forward, grab opponent, execute right front kick to knee...

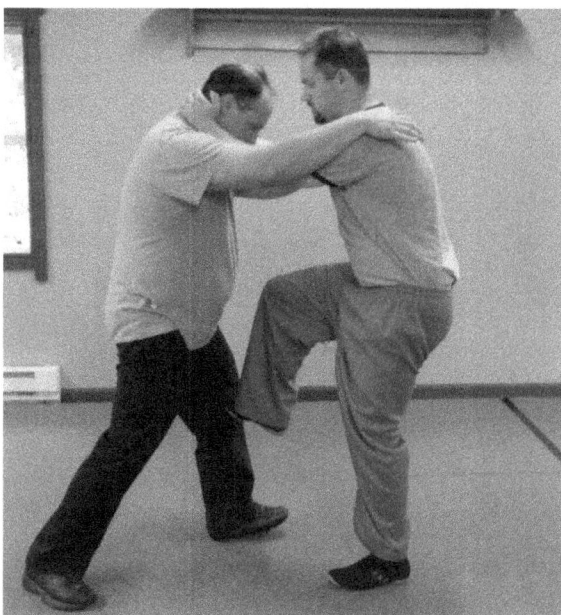

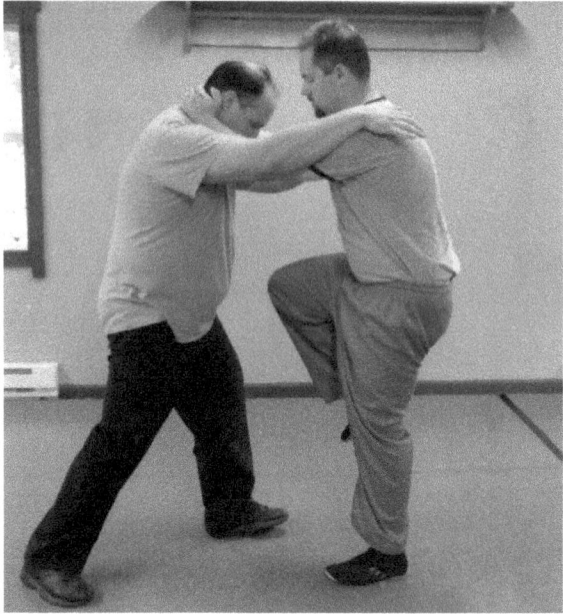

...follow up with right front knife edge kick to groin.

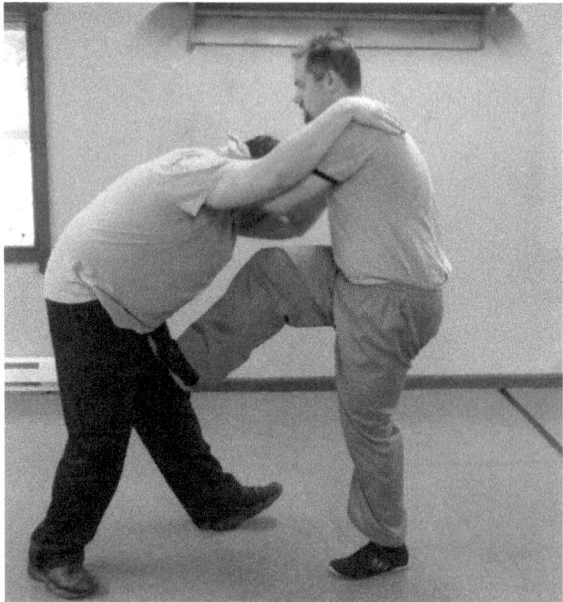

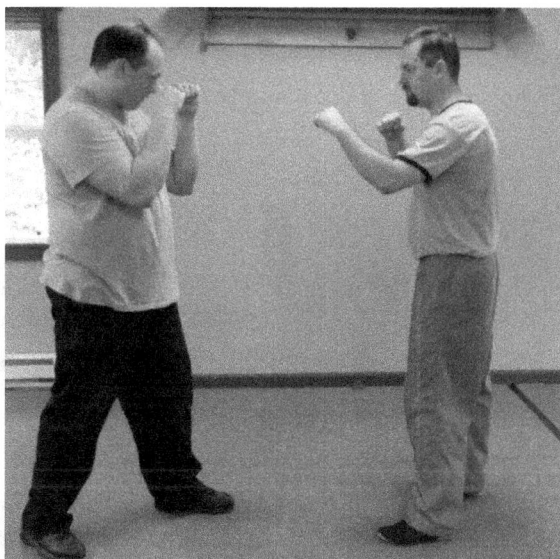

19. Facing opponent in left forward stance, both hands extended in guard position.

Forest Dragon Exercises

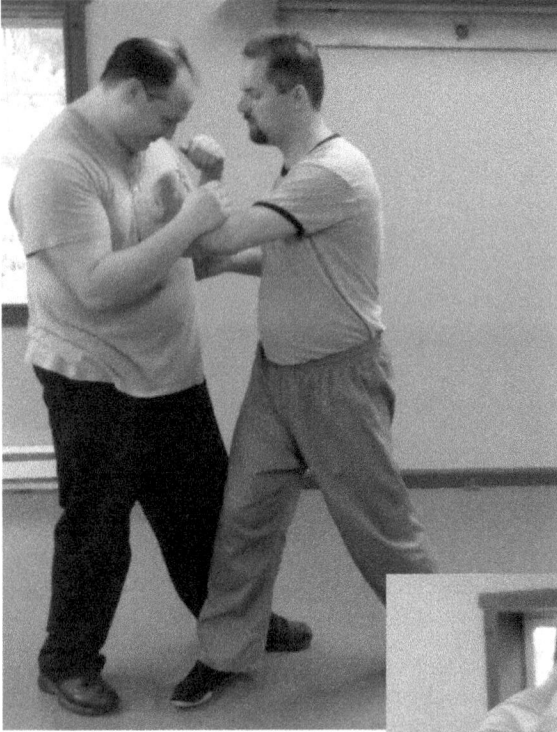

As soon as opponent approaches to attack, right foot steps forward into right forward stance extending left palm heel in short strike to chest.

Rear Angle:

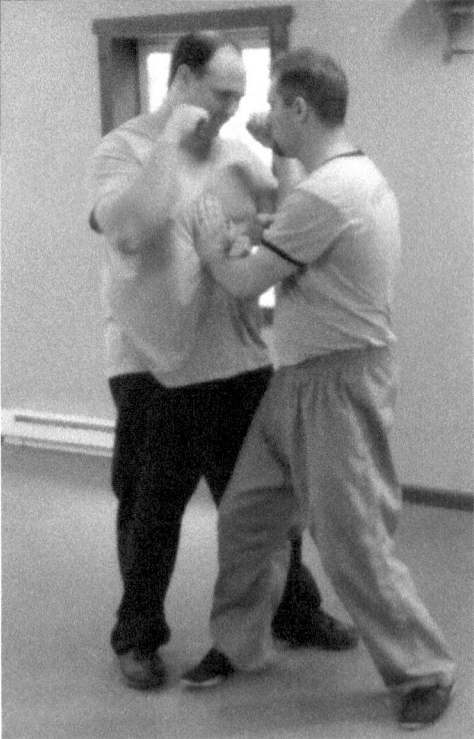

100

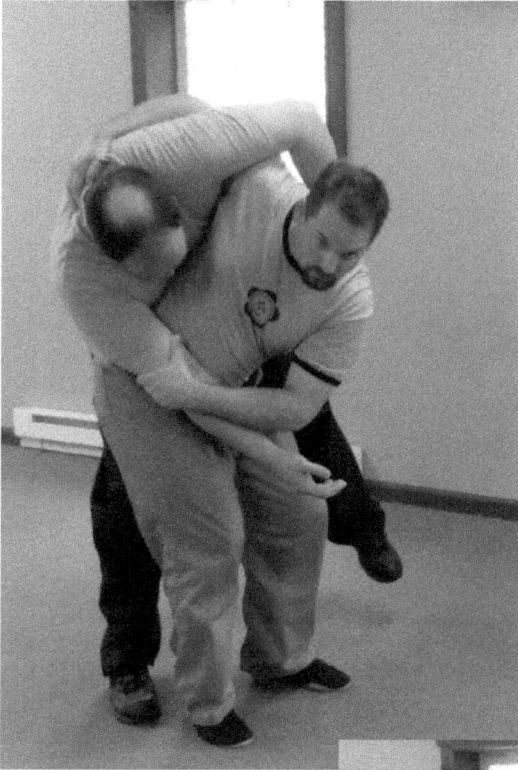

20. Turn 180° left while bringing left foot up next to right;

straighten legs, rising into attention stance, lifting opponent with hips.

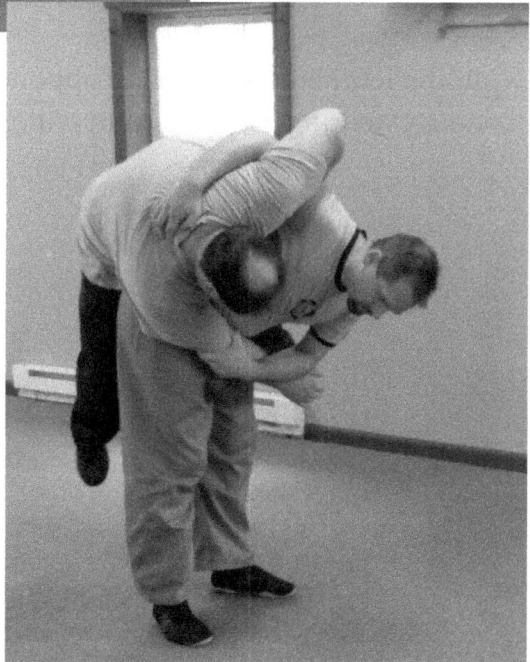

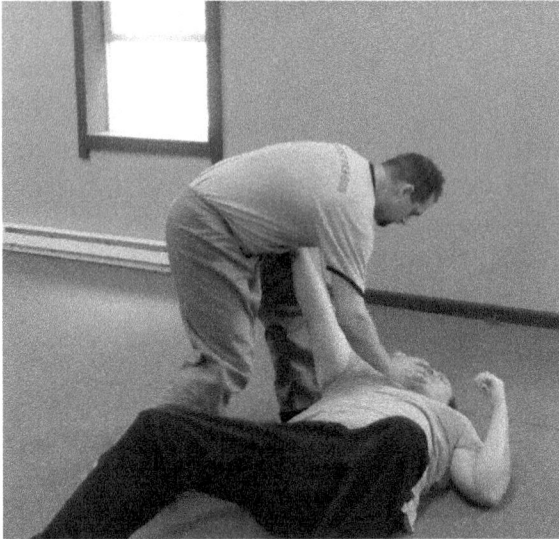

...pulling left hand back, bring opponent over hip and to the ground, extending right hand in willow leaf palm strike.

Daily Regimen

Forest Dragon Exercises

The Forest Dragon exercises are intended to provide a way for anyone to learn the fundamentals of Pai Lum while providing a means to a long and healthy life. One of the biggest challenges most people face is finding the time to practice. In the beginning of this book I said that the length of time a student practices is not as important as how often they practice. The goal should be to practice daily. I have provided an example of how a student can go through all of the exercises in this book in as little as ten minutes.

Begin with a simple minute or two of breathing meditation to clear the mind followed by five exercises to warm up the muscles and loosen up the joints. Continue by going through the movements of the Young Dragon form. There is no particular speed at which these should be done. Go as slow as necessary to do them correctly. This should only take about one minute. Going through the form twice will only take two minutes. End the session with another minute or two of breathing to replenish the body and relax the mind.

If you are able to spend more than ten minutes training, it is a simple matter of repeating some of the exercises. If possible, also spend more than two minutes doing the breathing and meditation. By setting a goal of training just ten minutes a day, you should find it easier to adhere to this regimen and with a little luck you will find yourself training more than ten minutes most days.

Forest Dragon Exercises

Daily Regimen

10 Minute Routine

Meditation

Earth Breathing   Circle Breathing   1-2 minutes

Qi Kung/Yoga

Heaven and Earth (Tadasana)	1 minute
Dancing Dragon (Natarajasana)	1 minute
Dragon Roll	1 minute
Head to Knee (Paschimottanasana)	1 minute
Dragon Boat (Navasana)	1 minute

Movement Form

Young Dragon   Earth   1-2 minutes

Meditation

Earth Breathing   Circle Breathing   1-2 minutes

Forest Dragon Exercises

Daily Regimen

30 Minute Routine

Meditation

Earth Breathing   Circle Breathing   5 minutes

Qi Kung/Yoga

Heaven and Earth (Tadasana)   2 minute
Dancing Dragon (Natarajasana)   2 minute
Dragon Roll   2 minute
Head to Knee (Paschimottanasana)   2 minute
Dragon Boat (Navasana)   2 minute

Movement Form

Young Dragon   Earth   10 minutes

Meditation

Earth Breathing   Circle Breathing   5 minutes

Forest Dragon Exercises

Closing Remarks

Forest Dragon Exercises

This book contains everything you need to get you started with the Forest Dragon exercises. I highly recommend finding a good teacher to guide you, especially if you are interested in the fighting aspects of the art. You can find a partial list of qualified Pai Lum teachers on the Forest Dragon web site.

Take the time to learn the exercises and to let your body learn the movements. Try not to rush. Many students are so eager to learn something new that they don't allow themselves to assimilate the techniques they already have. Repetition is important, but you also need to be mindful during your practice sessions.

I hope you find practicing these exercises enjoyable and that you will find them interesting. When you are comfortable with them you may want to begin the second book. In Phase II, you will be introduced to more breathing techniques, yoga exercises, and new concepts. This phase, represented by the Chinese element metal, is a refinement of the first phase, earth. It introduces new techniques and new ways to use the techniques you already have. The second phase takes the basic concepts and adds a new perspective to them and a different way of moving the body in a combat situation.

My last remark is to remind you of what my teacher was so fond of saying to me:

Practice!   Practice!   Practice!

And of course, remember to be mindful. But most of all...

"Have a good time!"

Forest Dragon Exercises

Appendix A – Rank in the Martial Arts

The martial arts ranking systems commonly used in the
United States are based on a system developed in Japan,
known as the Dan/Kyu system. The kyu, or lower grades, are
numbered from 9 to 1 (9th kyu being the lowest grade and 1st
kyu the highest). The dan ranks are the higher grades and
begin with the 1st dan (shodan in Japanese). The dan ranks are
recognizable by the black belt worn around the waist of the
traditional Japanese uniform or *gi*.

Many in the west regard a practitioner of 'black belt' status to
be a qualified instructor or expert. While wearing a black belt
conveys that the student has some level of proficiency,
reaching the 'black-belt' levels simply means that the
practitioner is a full-fledged student, no longer a beginner. In
many styles the title of teacher (*sensei* in Japanese styles, *shifu*
in Chinese styles) is not conferred until reaching a higher
rank, often fourth or fifth dan. In some systems the rank of
sensei may be independent of the dan rank of the practitioner,
being awarded based on the person's teaching ability and
maturity rather than solely on martial prowess. In most
systems a practitioner is at least a fourth higher level (fourth
dan or yondan in Japanese systems) before they are granted
the full unrestricted privileges of a teacher.

What is the highest rank one can attain in the martial arts?
Among the dan ranking of Japan, some systems allow for the
attainment of the 10th dan. Many of the traditional styles
allow 9th as the highest attainable rank, reasoning that 10th
dan signifies perfection, which is attainable only upon death.
Following this reasoning, some systems will confer the 10th
dan upon their most eminent upon death.

What Rank is a Master?

The term 'Master' is often surrounded by an aura of mysticism. To many it infers the notion of perfection.

In many styles the title of 'Master' may simply reflect the position that a teacher holds in his family or organization. He is the head of his school, just as we often say someone is "master of a household." Where appropriate, systems may have several masters all of whom are under the guidance, and authority, of a single Grand Master. *

Many students ask what it means to "be a good student". Often what they mean is how can I learn well and progress quickly. But there is a deeper, more traditional side to the question. Consider the following excerpt from the 17th century book written by a few samurai, "Ha Gakure" ("In the Shadow of Leaves"):

"A man is a good retainer to the extent that he earnestly places importance in his master. This is the highest sort of retainer. If one is born into a prominent family that goes back for generations, it is sufficient to deeply consider the matter of obligation to one's ancestors, to lay down one's body and mind, and to earnestly esteem one's master. It is further good fortune if, more than this, one had wisdom and talent and can use them appropriately. But even a person who is good for nothing and exceedingly clumsy will be a reliable retainer if only he has the determination to think earnestly of his master. Having only wisdom and talent is the lowest tier of usefulness."

* In many Chinese systems of martial arts teachers hold the title of *shifu* (pronounced sifu in Cantonese) which translates as teacher. There are two different words in Chinese which are pronounced "shifu", but the one typically used in the martial arts uses the Chinese character for father as the second syllable. Therefore the literal translation of shifu is "teacher-father".

116

One of the greatest threats to progressing in the martial arts is losing our humility. Some students think humility is about being treated poorly or having their rights suppressed in some way. Humility is actually quite simple; don't get so caught up in yourself that you become oblivious to everything and everyone around you. When I was still a beginner, having recently achieved my "green belt" and just become a Student Instructor, Li Lung was teaching a class on meditation. We were to concentrate on hearing and feeling our heartbeat. I remember him saying, "Practice until you can control your heart rate. Let me know when you can do that."

So I practiced diligently and soon was able to focus on relaxing and on getting my heart rate to slow down. I got one of the students in the school I was managing to check my pulse and confirmed that I wasn't just imagining it, I really could slow my heart rate. I was very impressed with myself. I thought, "Wow, I really am good. Li Lung will be very impressed with me." At the very next opportunity I told Li Lung of my great accomplishment and waited for an astonished look to come across his face.

Instead, he simply replied, "Good. Keep practicing."

Forest Dragon Exercises

Appendix B - Yoga

In ancient texts such as the Upanishads, yoga is described as composed of six branches (*sadanga*). In modern classical yoga the practice of yoga is categorized in eight steps or branches (*ashtanga*).

- Abstentions (yama)
- Observances (niyama)
- Postures (asana)
- Breath control/exercises (pranayama)
- Withdrawal of the senses (pratyahara)
- Fixed Attention (dharana)
- Meditation (dhyana)
- Concentration (samadhi)

The first five steps are considered external stages. The first two, abstentions and observances are considered preparation for the practice of yoga. Abstention includes such concepts as non-injury, truth, and non-possession. Observance puts forth rules for a "proper attitude" toward life, including purity and devotion. The next three steps develop control of the body, the breath, and the senses.

The postures, or asanas, are the physical movements and positions of the body which most people associate with yoga. These postures develop the muscular control of the body while focusing the mind.

Pranayama is the regulation and restraint of the breath. The systematic exercising of breath control helps bring the mind under control.

Pratyahara is the detachment of the senses. By reducing or shutting off the input of the senses, or five sources as they are often referred to in yoga, the stimulus to the mind is reduced allowing further relaxation. The remaining three steps are internal stages and considered "mind-control" exercises.

Dharana is the focusing of the mind on a particular point. The point of focus can be either internal such as the naval or center of the forehead, or external such as an object or point on the wall. Dhyana is the continuous and uninterrupted flow of thought, typically directed at a particular point, object, thought, or idea.

The eighth and final step of yoga is samadhi, or concentration. Concentration is the fully developed state of meditation. It is this state that is often referred to as a 'trance'. These last three steps in yoga when done at the same time are called samyama; that is, these last three techniques are directed toward the same object or thought simultaneously.

www.ingramcontent.com/pod-product-compliance
Lightning Source LLC
Chambersburg PA
CBHW060908280326
41934CB00007B/1228